Research and Relevance

Publications Committee of the
AMERICAN ACADEMY OF PSYCHOANALYSIS

Science and Psychoanalysis   Volume XXI

Research and Relevance

Scientific Proceedings of the
American Academy of Psychoanalysis

Edited by

JULES H. MASSERMAN, M.D.

Professor of Psychiatry and Neurology
Northwestern University, Chicago, Illinois

GRUNE & STRATTON   ·   New York and London

Grune & Stratton, Inc.
111 Fifth Avenue, New York, New York 10003

Library of Congress Catalog Card Number 58-8009
International Standard Book Number 0-8089-0768-9
Printed in the United States of America

Contents

Contributors

Aldrich, C. Knight, M.D., Professor and Chairman, Department of Psychiatry, New Jersey College of Medicine and Dentistry, Newark, New Jersey.

Alger, Ian, M.D., Clinical Assistant Professor of Psychiatry, New York Medical College, New York, New York.

Arieti, Silvano, M.D., Professor of Clinical Psychiatry, New York Medical College, New York, New York.

Bahnson, Claus B., Ph.D., Director, Department of Behavioral Sciences, Eastern Pennsylvania Psychiatric Institute, Philadelphia, Pennsylvania.

Brodie, H. Keith H., M.D., Assistant Professor, Department of Psychiatry, Stanford University, Palo Alto, California.

Chisholm, Shirley, Congresswoman, United States House of Representatives, from the 12th District of New York.

Chodoff, Paul, M.D., Clinical Professor of Psychiatry, George Washington University, Washington, D.C.

Dahlberg, Charles Clay, M.D., Training and Supervisory Analyst, William Alanson White Institute, New York, New York.

Epstein, Arthur W., M.D., Professor of Psychiatry and Neurology, Tulane University, School of Medicine, New Orleans, Louisiana.

Green, Maurice R., M.D., Research Psychiatrist and Training Analyst, William Alanson White Institute, New York, New York.

Gutierrez, Jose, M.D., Case Western Reserve University, Shaker Heights, Ohio.

Haar, Esther, M.D., Research Psychiatrist and Director of Division for Related Professions, William Alanson White Institute, New York, New York.

Havens, Leston L., M.D., Associate Clinical Professor of Psychiatry, Harvard Medical School, Boston, Massachusetts.

Hyams, Lyon, M.S., M.D., Director, Division of Biostatistics, Department of Community Medicine, Rutgers Medical School, New Brunswick, New Jersey.

Jaffe, Joseph, M.D., Chief of Psychiatric Research, New York State Psychiatric Institute, New York, New York.

Karno, Marvin, M.D., Department of Psychiatry, School of Medicine, University of California at San Diego, La Jolla, California.

Kelman, Harold, M.D., Dean, American Institute of Psychoanalysis, New York, New York.

Levy, Norman J., M.D., Attending Physician, University of New York Hospital, Brooklyn, New York.

Lifton, Robert Jay, M.D., Professor of Psychiatry, Yale University School of Medicine, New Haven, Connecticut.

Lipshutz, Daniel M., M.D., Research Psychiatrist, Public Schools, New York, New York.

Mandell, Arnold J., M.D., Professor and Chairman, Department of Psychiatry, School of Medicine, University of California at San Diego, La Jolla, California.

Markowitz, Irving, M.D., Medical Director, Family Service and Child Guidance Center of the Oranges, Maplewood and Millburn, East Orange, New Jersey.

Miller, Jean B., M.D., Clinical Assistant Professor of Psychiatry, Albert Einstein College of Medicine, New York, New York.

Miller, Susan E., R.N., Massachusetts Mental Health Center, Boston, Massachusetts.

Pierce, Chester M., M.D., Professor of Education and Psychiatry, Graduate School of Education, Harvard University, Cambridge, Massachusetts.

Reynolds, David, Ph.D., Assistant Professor (Anthropology), University of Southern California School of Medicine, Los Angeles, California.

Rubins, Jack L., M.D., Associate Clinical Professor of Psychiatry, New York Medical College; Director, Day-Care Center for Schizophrenia, Karen Horney Clinic, New York, New York.

Schechter, Marshall D., M.D., Professor of Psychiatry and Director, Division of Child Psychiatry, University of Oklahoma, Oklahoma City, Oklahoma.

Scheflen, Albert E., M.D., Professor of Psychiatry, Albert Einstein College of Medicine; Researcher at Bronx State Hospital and Jewish Family Service, New York, New York.

Strupp, Hans H., Ph. D., Professor of Psychiatry, Vanderbilt University, Nashville, Tennessee.

Tabachnick, Norman, M.D., Associate Chief Psychiatrist, Suicide Prevention Center; Clinical Professor of Psychiatry, University of Southern California, Los Angeles.

Taketomo, Yasuhiko, M.D., Career Scientist, New York Medical Center, New York, New York.

Ullman, Montague, M.D., Director, Department of Psychiatry, Maimonides Medical Center, Brooklyn, New York.

von Eckardt, Ursula M., Ph.D., School of Public Health, University of Puerto Rico, San Juan, Puerto Rico.

Will, Otto Allen, Jr., M.D., Director, Austen Riggs Center, Stockbridge, Massachusetts.

Wold, Carl I., Ph.D., Director of Research, Suicide Prevention Center; Assistant Clinical Professor of Psychiatry (Psychology), University of Southern California, Los Angeles, California.

Yamamoto, Joe, M.D., Professor of Psychiatry, University of Southern California School of Medicine, Los Angeles, California.

Preface to *Volume XXI and Requiem for*
Science and Psychoanalysis

Volume I of this series, entitled *Integrative Studies,* appeared in the spring of 1958 under the sponsorship of Dr. Henry M. Stratton, who, out of friendship for me and the fledgling American Academy of Psychoanalysis, agreed to assume the financial risk. The issue published our first scientific colloquium, with chapters by David M. Rioch, Percival Bailey, and Robert Heath on the biology of behavior, George Devereaux and Abraham Kardiner on anthropologic vectors, Jan Ehrenwald and Walter Reise on the pre-Freudian sources of psychoanalysis, Jurgen Ruesch, Sandor Rado, and Kenneth Appel on the dynamics of communication, Paul Hoch and Roy Grinker, Sr., on epistemologic considerations, James G. Miller on systems theory, a treatise on the psychodynamics of music and a memorial to Frieda Fromm-Reichmann by myself, and an appendix by Janet M. Rioch on the founding of the Academy. The seminar format thus initiated epitomized the Academy's scientific ideals: namely, to enrich analytic research, theory, and practice from the resources of other sciences and in turn offer them our own experiences and understandings. Subsequent volumes on ethology, family relationships, human values, cross-cultural studies, education, dreams, sexuality, marriage, violence, and on other fundamentals of the dynamics, vicissitudes, and therapy of human behavior contributed further to heuristic interdisciplinary integrations and merited highly favorable journal reviews, translations into several languages, and increasing acceptance as authoritative treatises throughout the world. The Academy thereby achieved the status of one of the most respected and scientifically influential organizations in its field.

I herewith wish to express my gratitude to the more than 300 authors who contributed to this success, and my appreciation to Grune & Stratton, who distributed the series internationally in an attractive format for permanent reference. However, since the Academy has decided to record its future proceedings in a quarterly periodical—an intrepid enterprise of which I declined the editorship—I must regretfully announce that this is the final volume of Science and Psychoanalysis, and wish the projected journal and its mentors every success.

JULES H. MASSERMAN, M.D.

Chicago, Illinois
June, 1972

part I

ONTOLOGY AND PHYSIOLOGY

Autism and Anaclitic Depression: Clinical Loci for a Counterintuitive Neurochemical Hypothesis

MARVIN KARNO, M.D.
ARNOLD J. MANDELL, M.D.

In a previous attempt to use neurochemical data to suggest heuristic phenomenological hypotheses, Mandell speculated that basic human affect states may represent the expressions of the interactions of three distinct neurochemical systems. These systems were seen as mediated by three specific neurotransmitter substances producing distinct forms of arousal or activation. Thus motor behavior, i.e., the general level of spontaneous activity, was postulated as a function of dopamine; methylated indoleamines, i.e., the methylated products of serotonin metabolism, were proposed as the transmission fuel of a "euphoria and creativity system"; and norepinephrine was considered the mediator of the degree of alertness or calm. [1]

The utility to the clinician and psychoanalytic theorist of such a "tripartite" rather than monoenergic notion of human affect is that it better corresponds to both everyday and clinical observations. In subjective life, the potential separateness of the components of affect are commonly experienced. Thus calm states of pleasant reverie and good feeling are conditions of elevation of mood without concomitant elevation of alertness or activity. On the other hand, a "really good day" may be blessed by a highly alert, pleasurable subjective state in the midst of a great deal of activity. When overtired, it is a common experience to feel motorically restless and alertly sensitive to stimulation while being subjectively dysphoric; that is, one can have the uncomfortable difficulty of "turning off" after a tiring experience. In the clinical arena, agitated depression is characterized by motor activation with simultaneous ruminative preoccupation, i.e., nonalertness to external cues, and a mood of persistent, internal pain and despair. Thus there is depression of mood and alertness but not of motor behavior. In contrast, retarded depressive states are characterized by *motor* retardation with variable degrees of dysphoric mood and reduced arousal. Reactive depressions, when not severe, may be characterized only by dysphoric mood with normal levels of activity and arousal. This would apparently be so even in the extreme case of the active, sociable individual who commits suicide and leaves behind a note indicative of a profound despair which was not revealed to his friends or family by his behavior or alertness.

In the following chapter Mandell proposes that affective states, and consequent adaptive behavior, may be subject to the more precise mediation of key enzymes in the biosyntheses of these three neurotransmitters, dopamine, norepinephrine, and serotonin. The enzymes tyrosine hydroxylase and tryptophan hydroxylase catalyze the hydroxylation of tyrosine to dopa, the immediate precursor to dopamine, which in turn is the immediate precursor of norepinephrine, and of tryptophan to 5-hydroxytryptophan, which is then decarboxylated to serotonin. A remarkable array of data has been presented in support of the extraordinary adaptational sensitivity via the fine tuning of the degree of activation and synthesis of these enzymes, in response to genetic, hormonal, pharmacologic, and environmental influences.[2]

The hypothesis is presented, using these data, that excitatory input in development or in adult experience may dampen the function of these neurotransmitter enzymes responsible for the maintenance of the various components of affect, and that input or environmental failure may lead to pathological activations of these systems. It is further proposed that a maladaptive, unregulated, i.e., out of feedback control, hyperactivation of this enzyme may underlie lasting states of depression, and that there may be important, other clinical ramifications to hereditary and environmental influences on this key enzyme's congenital base-line activity and subsequent vicissitudes in the individual's experience. For purposes of heuristic exercise in the synthesis of neurochemical speculation and clinical observation, we have chosen to consider briefly two forms of clearly defined and profound

psychiatric disturbance of earliest childhood, infantile autism and anaclitic depression. A review of some features of these childhood disorders
(as well as their experimentally induced animal analogues) will be considered in the light of these hypotheses.

Kanner, in his first report on the syndrome of infantile autism, emphasized that "the outstanding, 'pathognomic', fundamental disorder is
the childrens' *inability to relate themselves* in the ordinary way to people
and situations from the beginning of life. . . . there is from the start an
extreme autistic aloneness that, whenever possible, disregards, ignores,
shuts out anything that comes to the child from the outside. Direct physical
contact or such motion or noise as threatens to disrupt the aloneness is
either treated 'as if it weren't there', or if this is no longer sufficient, resented
painfully as distressing interference."[3]

Bergman and Escalona reported some years later on four psychotic
children whom they described as having been unusually and even extremely
sensitive to sensory stimulation, including change in equilibrium and
temperature, from very early in life. They postulated, using a concept of
Freud, that these children possessed a pathologically thin "protective
barrier" against stimulation, and that this ego deficiency may have been
influential in their development of psychosis.[4]

Fries and Woolf, several years later, described five categories of
infants, based on their congenital activity levels. These ranged from hypoactive to quiet to moderately active to active to hyperactive. They suggested
that such congenital activity types produce differential effects on parent-
child relationships, psychosexual development, ego development, defense
mechanisms, and predisposition to pathology. They believed that the
hypoactive and hyperactive infants were particularly vulnerable to the
development of psychopathology.[5]

Bettleheim, in a recent overview of infantile autism, expresses the
notion that the autistic child's apparent inattention to external stimulation
may be the product of excessive, repetitive, stereotyped self-stimulation.
He remarks that, through self-stimulation, ". . . outer stimuli are blotted
out by and 'lost' in the sensations the child stirs in himself. His own behavior
converts his state of 'wakefulness' into an overwhelming attentiveness to
himself and effectively obliterates his perception of reality."[6]

Bettleheim thus implies that the autistic child may be either supplying
or reinforcing his own "stimulus barrier" through self-stimulation which
serves as a competing or interfering shield against external stimuli.

Experiments in animal rearing have had the interesting result of
producing young animals which behave in ways very similar to autistic

children. Scott mentions two examples of such induced behavior. He describes the work of Kruijt,[7] who raised male jungle fowl in total isolation. As an adult, an isolation-reared fowl directs the ritual motions of courtship to his own body so that "... he spins and whirls in behavior never seen in ordinary roosters."[8] Self-spinning, repeated for long periods of time, has been reported as extremely common among autistic children. Studies by Fuller and Clark, as also recently described by Scott, have involved the rearing of dogs in isolation. A puppy, if isolated during a critical growth period, often displays "... bizarre postures such as standing still in the corner of a room with one paw raised above its head and forced into the angle of the walls."[9]

Scott mentions that an animal reared in isolation would be expected, from what we know of the process of primary socialization, to form an attachment, viz., to imprint itself on whatever is in its environment. This is apparently the case, for chickens reared in isolation behave as if they were imprinted on their own bodies. That such a narcissistic attachment may also characterize the autistic infant does not seem too remote a parallel.

The most provocative experimentation to date on the production of animal autism is the work of Harlow. Monkeys raised in isolation in bare wire cages displayed self-clutching and rocking movements early in life, idiosyncratic stereotypic and repetitive movements, and bizarre posturing. Harlow mentions that "an animal might sit in the front of its cage staring aimlessly into space. Occasionally one arm would slowly rise as if it were not connected to the body, and wrist and fingers would contract tightly—a pattern amazingly similar to the waxy flexibility characteristic of some human catatonic schizophrenics."[10]

What Kanner emphasized was the "painful resistance" of the autistic child to outside stimulation. Bergman and Escalona considered the supersensitivity to stimulation of some children as conducive to psychosis. Animal studies suggest that animals reared in isolation become hypercathected to the self as the source of stimulation, and Bettleheim suggests that autistic children may self-stimulatingly compete with and obliterate external stimuli.

The previously described chemical work has shown that rats maintained in relative sensory isolation develop an apparently compensatory increase in midbrain tyrosine hydroxylase; young chicks blinded in one eye similarly develop an apparently compensatory *increase* in the activity of the substance which mediates neurotransmission in the optic lobe serving that eye.[2] The apparently counterintuitive aspect of these findings is that the animals are apparently being neurochemically tuned to a higher level of responsivity in the face of decreased sensory input. That is, instead of a neurochemical disuse atrophy, there may be a disuse hypertrophy of baseline biosynthetic enzyme activity leading to the sensitization of some of the arousal systems described previously.

Assuming appropriate poetic license, we might speculate that the autistic child is normally in a state of sensory bombardment, its peculiar behavioral response to which may be correlated with a neurochemical detuning of biosynthetic enzyme activity. In other words, the autistic child might require an environment comparable to what we would consider a state of sensory deprivation in order to chemically tune up to the ordinary range of external input. Another way to see this is that the social or interpersonal pattern is a defense against the excruciating dysphoria of significant input amplified through sensitized arousal systems. This speculated situation is similar to that described by Bergman and Escalona[4] for their psychotic children. If this cycle of isolation to sensitization leading to more isolation is to be broken, one might predict a therapeutic response on the part of autistic children to relative sensory deprivation.

Such a response has in fact been recently reported by Schecter in the experimental treatment of 3 autistic children.[11] Schecter and his colleagues placed 2 boys of age 5 and 1 of age 4 in a specially designed room, for periods of 68, 74, and 40 days, respectively. The room provided minimum light, a constant low sound level, constant temperature, minimal human contact, and a minimum of inanimate objects.

Schecter has commented that "the research team postulated that the autistic defense is directed at overwhelming outer and inner stimuli. The defensive withdrawal is utilized repeatedly to cope with these stimuli and eventually becomes generalized to any and all stimuli. . . . Our team reasoned that an environment of sensory isolation would support these childrens' defenses and thereby decrease their need to use active withdrawal mechanisms constantly."[12]

The results, according to Schecter, were that "they [the children] were surprisingly content in the room and were able to drop many of the defenses that separated them from other people. They all made significant progress toward developing more satisfactory relationships with others, improved social and intellectual skills, and a better adjustment to their environments."[13] These very tentative but exciting clinical results suggest that the autistic child's response pattern may be able to be enduringly reset; i.e., his ego integrative capacity may be restructured through a specific kind of environmental experience, certainly consonant with many of the macromolecular theories of brain change with experience. The postulated neurochemical correlate, much more tentatively, is that the autistic child's pathologically detuned base line of biosynthetic enzyme activity may be reset to a more normal level by a carefully designed low sensory input environment. Of course, the new treatment procedure and its success, as is true of any new treatment procedure in psychiatry, must be interpreted with caution in view of the well-known Hawthorne effect of enthusiasm and special attention in experimental settings.[14]

Anaclitic depression during the second 6 mo. of life in institutionalized infants was of course first brought to wide attention by the classic reports of Spitz at the end of World War II.[15-17] Spitz reported that although the full-blown picture of anorexia, weight loss, weepiness, apathetic withdrawal, slowness, stupor, and insomnia was observed in only 19 of 123 children studied, another 26 children developed milder but recognizable symptoms. Provence and Lipton reported some years later on the dramatic affective differences in a group of 75 infants institutionalized since birth, in comparison with a matched group of family-reared infants. Their description is dramatic:

> They used no words, had no names for people or objects, and used very few vocal signals to express a feeling or to indicate a need. Their play with toys was impoverished, poorly elaborated, and repetitive; it lacked the signs of pleasure, interest and experimental zest seen in the family babies. . . . They seemed to have a low investment not only in all aspects of the environment but in themselves as well. . . . They had difficulty in being active either in order to make a contact to obtain comfort or pleasure or in order to avoid an unpleasant situation. They appeared virtually defenseless when faced with a painful stimulus.[18]

The more recent work of Harlow's group in inducing what they have called depression in young monkeys has produced remarkable analogues to anaclitic depression, both as originally defined by Spitz and as more recently summarized by Bowlby.[19] Harlow's group raised infant monkeys with their mothers and then separated the infants for periods of weeks. After an initial brief "protest" of increased vocalizing and motor activity, the monkeys apathetically withdrew, and became asocial and inactive. Harlow reports that essentially identical results of anaclitic depression in infant monkeys after maternal separation have been reported by two other primate laboratories.[20,21]

From our present focus of attention, we would postulate that normal infants, in the broad midrange of congenital activity type, present to their external environments with a midrange of neurochemical responsivity to stimulation. The withdrawal of a mothering companion apparently precipitates a sharp *decline* in responsivity which would presumably be corre-lated with the neurochemical event which our model predicts should be regularly present in the depressed states, viz., an increased level of midbrain tyrosine hydroxylase. The changes produced in animals with isolation produce precisely those enzymatic changes seen with chronic reserpine administration or in chronically hypothyroid animals—two chemical states well-known for producing the syndrome of "endogenous" depression in man.[2] This increased enzyme may be predicted to occur in response to the loss of the maternal input experience.

This temporary state is reversed abruptly by the reappearance of the mother, both in infant monkeys, according to Harlow, and in human infants, according to common clinical experience. Of course, prolonged or repeated separations produce more enduring abnormal states in the infant, presumably chemically as well as clinically.

The specificity of the mothering figure as the object maintaining a normal affect state in the infant may presumably be due to critical period learning of an imprinting and/or reinforcement nature. There would be apparent evolutionary adaptive value to having the totality of the infants cathexis of affect conditioned to the presenting mothering figure. We would then assume, similarly, a maternal conditioning of the neurochemical affective system.

In terms, then, of our admittedly highly simplified, premature, and tentative model, infantile autism and anaclitic depression may represent two expressions of the pathological sensitization of the biogenic amine system. The autistic child is in a state in which, given a high hereditary complement of enzymatic responsiveness, he needs to protect himself from input ampli-fication and thereby obtains temporary relief from isolation. The ana-clitically depressed infant, we propose, is in a state of (maternal) stimulus deprivation and elevated tyrosine hydroxylase activity leading to depressive or dysphoric affect. In this context, it is interesting that the tricyclic anti-depressants reduce midbrain tyrosine hydroxylase with the same kind of latency as their antidepressant effects in man.

On the basis of a recent finding that rat strains of varying base-line activity show base-line midbrain tyrosine hydroxylase activity levels inversely proportional to their motor activity levels,[22] we might speculate that infants who exhibit what Fries has described as a hypoactive con-genital activity type may similarly possess congenitally high biosynthetic enzyme activity levels. If this is so, we might predict that such infants would be "genetically prone" to the depressive experience. Thus these might be the children with potentially depressive ego structures.

We certainly have to enquire what it is that differentiated the infants who *did* develop anaclitic depression in Spitz's study from those who did not.

The depression-prone individual whom Rado many years ago described as "addicted to love" and whose deepest fixation point is the threat of loss of love[23] may well be the individual who is constitutionally suffering from a very thin buffer zone between normal base-line and clinically depressed levels of biosynthetic enzymatic activity. Thus such individuals might be those who respond quickly and profoundly to object loss. Indeed, the thickness of the ego's armor may reflect the thickness of the midbrain's chemical range between innate base-line activity and pathological response threshold.

References

1. Mandell, A. J.: Neurochemical considerations relevant to human affective states. In: Masserman, J. (Ed.): Depressions: Theories and Therapies, Vol. XVII of Science and Psychoanalysis. New York, Grune & Stratton, 1970.
2. Mandell, A. J., Segal, D. S., Kuczenski, R. T., and Knapp, S.: Some Factors in the Regulation of the Brain's Neurotransmitter Biosynthetic Enzymes and Receptor Sensitivity, Drug Mechanisms, and Behavior. Presented at the Symposium: Brain Chemistry and Behavior, UCSF, October 7, 1971, San Francisco, Calif.
3. Kanner, L: Autistic disturbances of affective contact. Nervous Child, 2:217–250, 1943.
4. Bergman, P., and Escalona, S. K.: Unusual sensitivities in very young children. Psychoanal. Stud. Child 3:4, 1947.
5. Fries, M. E., and Woolf, P. J.: Some hypotheses on the role of the congenital activity type in personality development. Psychoanal. Stud. Child 8–62, 1953.
6. Bettleheim, B.: Infantile autism. In Arieti, S. (Ed.): The World Biennial of Psychiatry and Psychotherapy, Vol. 1. New York, Basic Books, 1971, p. 418.
7. Scott, J. P.: Early Experience and the Organization of Behavior. Belmont, Calif., Wadsworth Publishing Co., 1968.
8. Kruijt, J. P.: Ontogeny of Social Behavior in Burmese Red Jungle Fowl. Leiden, Brill, 1964.
9. Fuller, J. L., and Clark, L. D.: Genetic and treatment factors modifying the post-isolation syndrome in dogs, J. Comp. Physiol. Psychol. 61:251–257, 1966a.
10. Harlow, H. F., Harlow, M. K., and Suomi, S. J.: From thought to therapy: Lessons from a primate laboratory. Amer. Sci. 59:538–549, 1971.
11. Schecter, M. D., Shurley, J. T., Toussieng, D. W., et al: Sensory isolation therapy of autistic children: A preliminary report. J. Pediat. 74:564–569, 1969.
12. *Ibid.*, p. 565.
13. *Ibid.*, p. 569.
14. Shapiro, A. K.: The placebo effect in medicine, psychiatry and psychotherapy. In: Bergin, A. E., and Garfield, S. (Eds.): Handbook of Psychotherapy and Behavior Change: An Empirical Analysis. New York, Wiley, 1971.

15. Spitz, R. A.: Hospitalism, Psychoanal. Stud. Child 1:53–74, 1945.
16. Spitz, R. A.: Hospitalism, a follow-up report. Psychoanal. Stud. Child 2:113–117, 1946.
17. Spitz, R. A.: Anaclitic depression. Psychoanal. Stud. Child 2:313–342, 1946.
18. Provence, S., and Lipton, R. C.: Infants in Institutions. New York, International Universities Press, 1962, p. 160.
19. Bowlby, J.: Attachment and Loss. Vol. I: Attachment. New York, Basic Books, 1969.
20. Kaufman, I. C. and Rosenblum, L. A.: The reaction to separation in infant monkeys: Anaclitic depression and conservation withdrawal. Psychosom. Med. 29:648–675, 1967.
21. Hinde, R. A., Spencer-Booth, Y., and Bruce, M.: Effects of 6-day maternal deprivation on rhesus monkeys, Nature 210:1021–1033, 1966,
22. Segal, D. S., Kuczenski, R. T., and Mandell, A. J.: Strain differences in behavior and brain tyrosine hydroxylase activity. Behav. Biol., 1971. In press.
23. Rado, S.: The Problem of melancholia. Int. J. Psychoanal. 9:420–437, 1928.

Isolation and Neurochemical Sensitization—A Counterintuitive Hypothesis

ARNOLD J. MANDELL, M.D.

MARVIN KARNO, M.D.

If one were to take a hard look at the source of hypotheses, the processes of their explication, and their validation in the metapsychological writing of psychoanalysis, one would have to conclude that the intuitive process plays a most significant role. A self-examination while reading metapsychological articles about such issues as psychic energy, states of consciousness, a theory of affect, and child development would probably reveal one's mind turning to a symphony of clinical memories, existential subjective feelings, and a gradually definable intuitive grasp of the author's message that had both cognitive and feeling elements. One either "becomes convinced" or fails to "become convinced." In this process dominated by subjectivity, some writers exploit their capacity to deal with what one might call "resistances" or exploit the presold acceptability of their reputation and image (i.e., preexisting transference). The next clinical or human experience that one has that brings to mind the new concept leads to the enrichment of the new percept and the continuation of a process that leads to the gradual institution of the metapsychological construct into the conceptual armamentarium of the clinician. Very often, of course, these intuitively derived and validated metapsychological constructs can be taken to other arenas for tests such as nursery schools, surveys of large clinical populations, or clinical psychoanalytic situations. Numerous meetings, discussions, and seminars lead to the gradual shaping of a common metapsychological language made out of a collection of these intuitively derived metapsychological constructs. This intellectual sharing is often the interpersonal and social matrix around which such processes occur.

When such processes involving metapsychological theory are addressed by those concerned with social science epistemology, they are often characterized as "unscientific". . . usually by implication. On the other hand, metapsychologicalizing, when presented as growing out of the context of clinical data, has been defined as the scientific method of psychoanalysis. If this issue is debated (and it seldom is anymore), it usually becomes one in which attempts are made to examine whether in fact the metapsychological concepts are expressed in ways which can be operationalized and subjected to tests—clinical or otherwise. Such discussions, although aiding practitioners with definitions of terms, seldom are taken to other arenas, seldom are tested in arenas dominated by data from convergent sources. The relationship between the model and the data becomes an epistemological exercise in which the value or belief systems of the people involved so heavily dominate that, very often if not always, discussions are nonproductive. A typical question that dominates such a discussion is whether behaviors in apparent logical opposition could be interpreted as metapsychologically identical.

Anyone whose own particular heritage has included some psychoanalytic training as well as brain biology must be more tolerant of the metapsychologist owing to the fact that in both games of science where human behavior is concerned, there is a long distance between theory and data. As a matter of fact, one could say that the current state of the art in behavioral neuropharmacology or neurochemistry has very little to teach metapsychologists with perhaps one very important exception, an example of which we hope to present here. Forrester in his recent book on complex social systems has demonstrated that systems in trouble manifest solutions to their problems and explanations of themselves which of course are a function of the system.[1] In more practical terms, he points out that if one is looking for a solution to problems in a system, very often the solutions that are being offered by the system itself are manifestations of the same problem. More housing in the ghetto neighborhood to produce a bigger ghetto is one of his examples. In this same way one can conceive of our intuitive explanations of our own brain functions based on our relationship to ourselves and others as being a reflection of the operations of the system. In the practice of psychoanalysis we almost routinely retreat from the assumptions and operations extant in our patient's free associations. We do what in fact we call "look below" the overt content. We use many techniques and concepts to do this but probably most importantly, productions of our own cognitive and unconscious mind which at some level are not consonant with the system with which we are being presented. This disjunction or alienation of associative processes makes it possible for us to begin to derive assumptions which from the standpoint of the patient-free associator might be viewed as counterintuitive; that is, inconsonant with his current system of assumptions and operations. The metapsychological theorist, however, is in a bind. He has no position from which to receive this experience of disjunction or alienation vis-à-vis his internal process during the generation of theoretical models. As a matter of fact, one might say that almost by necessity his theoretical model can only be a manifestation of his own internal cognitive and subjective system.

In previous papers the senior author has outlined the various functions of such theory building as an aid to doing clinical work.[2] Purer metapsychological theorizing directed toward the understanding of human behavior has more diffuse goals. Allen Wheelis, in his novels portraying a progressively more cynical and nihilistic psychoanalyst, has portrayed metapsychological theory building as a way of creating a national reputation and lucrative practice.[3] Lest such sacrilegious thoughts be seen as exclusive in the domain of bitter psychoanalysts, one is reminded of Irving Page's description of the major function of serotonin which was "to afford tenure to Pharmacology Professors."[4] It is my feeling that the enrichment of the perceptions of human behavior by metapsychological theorists is the major contribution in this area. Their work often leads to varying kinds of research both psychoanalytic and otherwise, but almost always to the enrichment of the associations and transactional comfort of the practicing clinician.

The major contribution of neuropharmacology and neurochemistry to such metapsychological theories has seemed to us to be as a source of counterintuitive hypotheses; that is, as an alien system from which vantage point more indigenous thoughts and ideas can arise. This chapter has as its goal the description of some work leading to what we would call a counterintuitive set. The chapter which precedes this one ties together in a rich and varigated way issues of animal, human, and clinical behavior in which such a counterintuitive hypothesis might be useful. Dr. Marshall Schecter perhaps has already used our counterintuitive hypothesis in his clinical research.

Stated in its most simple terms, the counterintuitive hypothesis goes something like this: In terms of the brain tissue subsuming such organismic states as elation, depression, anger, sexuality, tension, attention, and calm, and relating function to structural change, *the brain is unlike a muscle.* In terms of relating use to preparation for use, much elegant work has demonstrated that exercise produces muscle hypertrophy. Increases in enzymatic mechanisms relating to muscle contraction following use have been documented.[5] We wish to present evidence that the subcortical biogenic amine systems when used extensively turn off. When used minimally, they hypertrophy.

The commonest way to relate neurochemistry to behavior in man currently is by relating the neurochemistry of the drug effect in animal brains to the behavioral effect of the drug in man. The assumption underlying what Schildkraut has called "the pharmacological bridge"[6] is that in the primitive areas of animal brains, neurochemical alterations produced by drugs are probably similar to those produced by drugs in man. Another assumption underlying this work is that the drug-induced behavioral manifestations in man due to the complexity of the human brain may make it difficult or impossible to relate these effects to behavioral changes in animals. Using this approach, the biological parameters have been drug effects on synaptic levels of neurotransmitters. More specifically, various drugs influencing the biogenic amine systems were supposed to function by increasing or decreasing available neurotransmitters to receptors in the subcortical brain systems subsuming organismic states such as mood, motility, anger, sexuality, and anxiety. The specific synaptic process that has been emphasized is the process of uptake and release of neurotransmitters. Drugs like Tofranil function by blocking reuptake catecholamines making more catecholamines available to the synapse and therefore improving mood.[6] Figure 1 demonstrates a summary of a wide variety of drug mechanisms as classically conceived. As one can see, the availability of synaptic neurotransmitter is emphasized as the important intervening variable in producing drug effects.

The work of several laboratories including ours in recent years,[7-10] however, has demonstrated that in active neural systems, newly synthesized rather than stored neurotransmitter is the synaptically active fraction. That is, the presynaptic neuron appears to make neurotransmitter as it is needed. It has thus become very important to describe and characterize the regulation of the neurotransmitter biosynthetic apparatus in the presynaptic neuron. As we have recently reviewed,[11,12] there are many exquisite regulators for such synthetic activity allowing wide variation

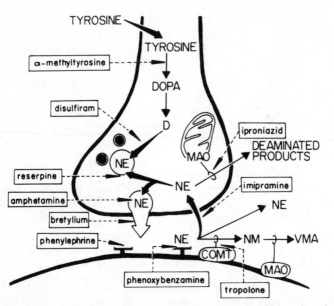

Fig. 1. The commonest model of the noradrenergic synapse in which various drugs are shown to influence synthesis, storage, release, reuptake, and degradation of noradrenaline. NE = norepinephrine, MAO = monoamine oxidase, D = dopamine, DOPA = dihydroxyphenylalanine, COMT = catechol-O-methyltransferase, NM = normetanephrine, and VMA = 3-methoxy-4-hydroxymandelic acid. Note that the biosynthetic process is shown as replenishing the storage form of the catecholamines with the other mechanisms more involved with synaptic events.

in the degree, latency, and duration of enzyme modulation. Some of these mechanisms are summarized in Fig. 2. One of the measures, however, that we have used consistently and interestingly to relate to behavior has been the activity level of the critical biosynthetic enzymes. The critical role these enzymes play may be visualized in the following way: Imagine a number of enzymes in a row like a production line; the rate of production would be determined by the slowest step. This slowest-step enzyme, then (the amount or degree of activity of it), appears to determine the rate of function of a chemically defined neural system. To put it in another graphic way, if there is a huge crowd trying to get through the doorway, the size of the doorway determines how many people are getting through. Since in the brain things happen so very quickly, it is hard to count the people getting through the doorway (molecules of neurotransmitter impinging on a receptor); it is relatively easy to measure the size of the doorway

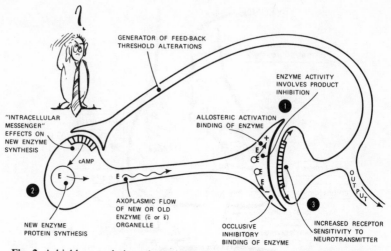

GENERATOR OF FEED-BACK
THRESHOLD ALTERATIONS

ENZYME ACTIVITY
INVOLVES PRODUCT
INHIBITION

"INTRACELLULAR
MESSENGER"
EFFECTS ON
NEW ENZYME
SYNTHESIS

ALLOSTERIC ACTIVATION
BINDING OF ENZYME

cAMP

AXOPLASMIC FLOW
OF NEW OR OLD
ENZYME (ē or s̄)
ORGANELLE

NEW ENZYME
PROTEIN SYNTHESIS

OCCLUSIVE
INHIBITORY
BINDING OF ENZYME

INCREASED RECEPTOR
SENSITIVITY TO
NEUROTRANSMITTER

OUTPUT

Fig. 2. A highly speculative scheme integrating some of the adaptive mechanisms of neurotransmitter biosynthetic enzymes under study in our laboratory. 1 signifies the binding activation and/or occlusion of nerve terminal, neurotransmitter biosynthetic enzymes in response to changes in intraneuronal, extravesicular biogenic amine concentration. 2 represents the reception of the feedback of information from the postsynaptic cell to the presynaptic cell body that regulates new enzyme protein synthesis (or degradation) followed by axoplasmic flow of new enzyme to the terminals where it is appropriately bound. 3 indicates the postsynaptic area which we have evidence has the capacity to develop increases in sensitivity following presynaptic denervation or treatment. Here regulation of biosynthesis is emphasized as the critical modulator of synaptic transmitter.

(the amount or activity of the rate-limiting enzyme). Critical neurotransmitter biosynthetic enzymes, seen either as the slow step in a production line or the doorway in a crowd exit, are our measure of the synthesis rate of a neurotransmitter. We have related these biosynthetic enzyme levels with various circumstances but the one we will describe to you today has to do with the interesting relationship that exists between this measure and indices of general input from the environment and activity level.

Figure 3 represents the results of two experiments in which newborn White Leghorn chicks were blinded on one side at birth. Because their optic tracts completely decussate without mixing, the input from one eye goes completely over to the opposite optic lobe. Thus, by blinding one eye at birth one produces a "blind" lobe and a "seeing" lobe for comparison. The animals were sacrificed 2 wk. after birth. Note that although the differences do not quite reach significance, both experiments show the

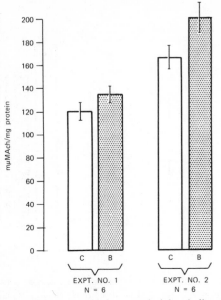

Fig. 3. The effect of enucleation at birth on optic lobe choline acetyltransferase activity in the newborn chick. C are the lobes opposite the good eye. B are the lobes opposite the blinded eye.

trend in which with blinding there is an increase in the acetylcholine-synthesizing enzyme in the opposite optic lobe. That is, with a *decrease* in input during development, the chick's optic lobe neurotransmitter biosynthetic apparatus hypertrophies. Figure 4 demonstrates another experiment relating input to enzymatic capacity in which if the animals are treated with amphetamine daily (which we conceive of as stimulating brainstem input to the optic lobes) the denervation hypertrophy is somewhat modified. Recent studies[13] of neurotransmitter biosynthetic enzymes in rats isolated alone in dark rooms compared to rats maintained in groups for 4, 8, and 16 days demonstrated a similar relative increase in tyrosine hydroxylase in the midbrain and caudate of the isolated rats. Figure 5 demonstrates these changes in the enzyme responsible for the biosynthesis of norepinephrine and dopamine. It is of interest that the activity of the nerve-ending serotonin biosynthetic enzyme tryptophan hydroxylase decreases. If one is to accept the premise that norepinephrine and dopamine are activating transmitters and serotonin a sedating one, it appears as though once again we are confronted with the circumstance of a markedly decreased input

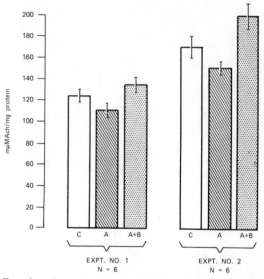

Fig. 4. The effect of amphetamine and blinding on the specific activity of chick brain, optic lobe choline acetyltransferase in the newborn chick. The chicks are enucleated at birth and treated with amphetamine. C are the saline-treated control animals. A are the amphetamine-treated animals. A and B are lobes from blinded animals treated with amphetamine, 10 mg. b.i.d.

leading to the subcortical biogenic amine system response leading to hyperactivity. If one wished to view the grouped animals as an experimental group, one might then interpret the experiment the other way in which high input produced lower levels of neurotransmitter biosynthetic enzyme. Tables 1A, 1B, and 1C are a summary of data relating spontaneous motor and exploratory behavior in five rat strains with the neurotransmitter biosynthetic enzyme tyrosine hydroxylase. Here too, one sees an interesting and important inverse relationship between the enzyme producing the so-called activating neurotransmitters and motor activity. We have thus far assumed that the genetic component leading to the behavior is at some third place influencing neurotransmitter biosynthetic enzymes and behavior. Once again one sees that under circumstances of potentially high synaptic activity one decreases the enzyme complement and vice versa.

The counterintuitive hypothesis for which evidence is presented says that even in such a general system as the arousal system, sensitization occurs in isolation and desensitization in high input states. Work recently done by Welch[14] demonstrated the marked increase in sensitization to the

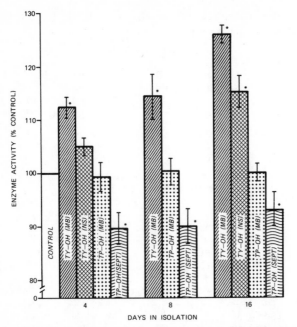

Fig. 5. The effect of isolation of rats in a sound-attenuated darkened room for 4, 8, and 16 days on midbrain (MB), neostriatal (NS), and septal (SEPT) tyrosine hydroxylase (TY-OH) and tryptophan hydroxylase (TP-OH) activities. Note that there is an immediate and progressive increase in midbrain tyrosine hydroxylase, and delayed increase in neostriatal tyrosine hydroxylase, and an immediate decrease in septal tryptophan hydroxylase.

toxic effects of amphetamine in animals kept in isolation before treatment. This finding is consonant with our observed changes in tyrosine hydroxylase. It would seem to me that "input shutdown" or "isolation sensitization" may have interesting phenomenological implications for the clinician and metapsychological theorist. Although consonant with some previous behavioral observations and theories, it would suggest a counterintuitive orientation particularly in reference to the components of metapsychology dealing with the reception, storage, and discharge of input. The critical role "excitation management" has played in the derivation of both the structural and energetic models of psychoanalytic theory, particularly of development, becomes less than immediately acceptable as one abandons the reflex arc as a space-limited warehouse of input and begins to see an input-triggered dampening mechanism as significant. Even open social

Table 1. Strain Differences in Levels of Tyrosine Hydroxylase and Spontaneous Activity

A. *Spontaneous Activity*

Strain		BUF	SD	LEW	ACI	BN	F344
		137*	121	114	92	59	46
		± 29	± 27	± 24	± 29	± 15	± 4
		($n = 7$)	($n = 7$)	($n = 7$)	($n = 7$)	($n = 7$)	($n = 7$)
BUF	137 ± 29	—	—	—	—	—	—
SD	121 ± 27	N.S.	—	—	—	—	—
LEW	114 ± 24	N.S.	N.S.	—	—	—	—
ACI	92 ± 29	N.S.	N.S.	N.S.	—	—	—
BN	59 ± 15	< 0.01	< 0.05	< 0.05	N.S.	—	—
F344	46 ± 4	< 0.01	< 0.001	< 0.001	< 0.05	N.S.	—

B. *Striatal Tyrosine Hydroxylase*

Strain		BUF	SD	LEW	BN	ACI	F344
		12485†	13919	14867	15079	15572	17944
		± 556	± 406	± 265	± 982	± 902	± 418
		($n = 10$)	($n = 15$)	($n = 15$)	($n = 5$)	($n = 10$)	($n = 15$)
BUF	12485 ± 556	—	—	—	—	—	—
SD	13919 ± 406	< 0.01	—	—	—	—	—
LEW	14867 ± 265	< 0.001	< 0.01	—	—	—	—
BN	15079 ± 982	N.S.	N.S.	N.S.	—	—	—
ACI	15572 ± 902	< 0.01	< 0.05	N.S.	N.S.	—	—
F344	17944 ± 418	< 0.001	< 0.001	< 0.001	< 0.05	< 0.002	—

C. *Midbrain Tyrosine Hydroxylase*

Strain		BUF	ACI	SD	LEW	BN	F344
		1596†	1707	1830	1831	2432	2613
		± 139	± 75	± 122	± 120	± 100	± 66
		($n = 4$)	($n = 10$)	($n = 15$)	($n = 10$)	($n = 5$)	($n = 5$)
BUF	1596 ± 139	—	—	—	—	—	—
ACI	1707 ± 75	N.S.	—	—	—	—	—
SD	1830 ± 122	N.S.	N.S.	—	—	—	—
LEW	1831 ± 120	N.S.	N.S.	N.S.	—	—	—
BN	2432 ± 100	< 0.004	< 0.001	< 0.01	< 0.01	—	—
F344	2613 ± 66	< 0.004	< 0.001	< 0.01	< 0.001	N.S.	—

Levels of significance were calculated using the Mann-Whitney U test (Siegel, 1957).

*Mean number of crossovers ± S.E.M.

†Mean cpm/20 min./mg. protein ± S.E.M.

system models emphasizing unique cognitive and symbolic meanings have not excaped from the premise that input of excitation leads to an expanded capacity, inclination, or impulse for discharge—the work presented here may lead to another look.

References

1. Forrester, J. M.: Urban Dynamics. Cambridge, Massachusetts Institute of Technology Press, 1969.
2. Mandell, A. J.: Theory building—A treatment for the therapist of schizophrenics. J. Nerv. Ment. Dis. 25:1–4, 1964.
3. Wheelis, A.: The Quest for Identity. New York, Norton Press, 1958.
4. Page, I.: Serotonin (5-hydroxytryptophan); the last 4 years. Physiol. Rev. 38:277–335, 1958.
5. Kielley, W. W.: The biochemistry of muscle. Ann. Rev. Biochem. 33:403–430, 1964.
6. Schildkraut, J. J.: The pharmacological bridge. In: Mandell, A. J., and Mandell, M. P. (Eds.): Psychochemical Research Strategies in Man. New York, Academic Press, 1969, pp. 113–126.
7. Weiner, N.: Regulation of norepinephrine biosynthesis. Ann. Rev. Pharmacol. 1970.
8. Dairman, W., and Udenfriend, S.: Increased conversion of tyrosine to catecholamines in the intact rat following elevation of tissue tyrosine hydroxylase levels by administered phenoxybenzamine. Molec. Pharmacol. 6:360–366, 1970.
9. Mueller, R. A., Thoenen, H., and Axelrod, J.: Inhibition of transsynaptically increased tyrosine hydroxylase activity by cycloheximide and actinomycin D. Molec. Pharmacol. 5:463–469, 1969.
10. Mandell, A. J., Segal, D. S., Kuczenski, R. T., and Knapp, S.: Some factors in the regulation of the brain's neurotransmitter biosynthetic enzymes and receptor sensitivity, drug mechanisms and behavior. In: McGaugh, J. (Ed.): Brain Chemistry and Behavior, 1972. In press.
11. Kuczenski, R. T., and Mandell, A. J.: Allosteric activation of hypothalamic tyrosine hydroxylase by ions and sulfated mucopolysaccharides. J. Neurochem., 1971. In press.
12. Segal, D. S., Sullivan, J. L., Kuczenski, R. T., and Mandell, A. J.: Effects of long-term reserpine treatment on brain tyrosine hydroxylase and behavioral activity. Science 173:842–843, 1971.
13. Segal, D. S., Kuczenski, R. T., Knapp, S., and Mandell, A. J.: Isolation and neurotransmitter biosynthetic enzyme activity. In preparation.
14. Welch, B. L., and Welch, A. S.: Control of brain catecholamines and serotonin during acute stress and after d-amphetamine by natural inhibition of monoamine oxidase: An hypothesis. In: Costa, E., and Garattini, S. (Eds.): The Amphetamines. 1970, pp. 415–446.

Discussion by H. Keith H. Brodie, M.D.

To base a theory on 12 chickens, all of which were half-blind, seems a bit preposterous, yet I believe Dr. Mandell has proposed a useful model of isolation sensitization.

Dr. Mandell is relating environmental input and activity levels to brain enzyme activity. His principal thesis is that increased neuronal activity, as reflected by an increase in input over the visual system or by an increase in output as measured by spontaneous activity, is associated with a decrease in those brain enzymes which regulate the synthesis of certain neurotransmitters. He is persuading us that the brain is not like a muscle, but is rather like a battery which, with use, decreases with activity, but, on resting, chemically regains its charge.

Other investigators have shown that a decrease in visual stimulation, through either blinding or environmental manipulation, causes several changes in the occipital cortex of rats, the most significant of which are a diminished electrical response, a decrease in the size and weight of the occipital cortex, a decrease in the number of dendritic spines, and increases in enzyme activity, the most dramatic being a 7 percent increase in acetylcholinesterase.[1] This last finding certainly supports Dr. Mandell's hypothesis.

Methodologically, Dr. Mandell's work has some weaknesses. I am concerned about the data on choline acetyltransferase both in the enucleation experiment and in the enucleation-plus-amphetamine experiment. The differences between enzyme activities in these two experiments are not statistically significant. Perhaps a larger *n* would yield significance. It is reassuring to see stars on the isolation stress figure, possibly indicating statistical significance has been reached; nonetheless it would be good to know the level of significance as well as the number of animals used in this experiment. One wonders what happened to tyrosine hydroxylase in the caudate after 8 days of isolation. These data were not recorded on the graph.

Dr. Mandell's theory has certain clinical applications, some of which Drs. Karno and Schecter will be discussing. I would like to present data on the treatment of depression using alpha-methyl-para-tyrosine (AMPT), an inhibitor of tyrosine hydroxylase, the enzyme which Dr. Mandell has described to you as the rate-limiting enzyme in catecholamine synthesis.[2] Now if retarded depression is associated with an increase in tyrosine hydroxylase, which we would expect from Dr. Mandell's theory, then AMPT should be an effective treatment for retarded depression.

Our initial series of 3 patients hospitalized for retarded depression were given up to 4 gm. of AMPT daily on a double-blind basis over the course of 2 wk. Although this dose was effective in decreasing the concentration of the dopamine metabolite homovanillic acid in the cerebrospinal fluid, and in increasing REM time, it was not effective in treating depression. In fact, it made our patients worse. Recently Bunney has expanded this series to include 10 depressed patients, none of whom showed improvement on AMPT.[3]

These data refute the Mandell hypothesis clinically. I might suggest, however, that Dr. Mandell may be correct if he relates depression to brain hyperactivity rather than hypoactivity. Then depression would be associated with a deficit of tyrosine hydroxylase and should become worse following treatment with the tyrosine hydroxylase inhibitor.

In summary, we have been presented with a fine sample of metapsychology as applied to brain biology. I would hope that Dr. Mandell continues his work, that it reaches statistical significance, and that perhaps Dr. Mandell should modify his view of depression to include brain hyperactivity. I hope that in the months ahead the distance between the Mandell theory and the data becomes shorter. I feel confident that it will have served a useful model in our understanding of affective disorders.

References

1. Rosenzweig, M. R.: Effects of environment on development of brain and behavior. In: Tobach, E. (Ed.): Biopsychology of Development. New York, Academic Press, 1971, pp. 303–342.
2. Brodie, H. K. H., Murphy, D. L., Goodwin, F. K., and Bunney, W. E., Jr.: Catecholamines and mania: The effect of alpha-methyl-para-tyrosine on manic behavior and catecholamine metabolism. Clin. Pharmacol. Ther. 12:218–224, 1971.
3. Gershon, E. S., Bunney, W. E., Jr., Goodwin, F. K., Murphy, D. L., Dunner, D. L., and Henry, G. M.: Catecholamines and affective illness: Studies with L-DOPA and alpha-methyl-para-tyrosine. In: Ho, B. T., and McIsaac, W. M. (Eds.): Brain Chemistry and Mental Disease. New York, Plenum Press, 1971, pp. 135–162.

Discussion by Marshall D. Schechter, M.D.

Throughout the history of science construction of hypotheses and paradigms has preceded practical applications. In psychiatric explorations there have been consistent attempts to move from macroscopic observations to microscopic explanations with interventions appropriately and properly based on the considered models. Inherent in each of these constructions has been the utilization of the intuitive process in the observer who at times confirms the correctness of his views by a potentially self-fulfilling prophecy. The results are more apt to be preconditioned especially in those model makers who come into the experimental situation with a preformed theory and conscious and/or unconscious mental bibliographic references. More often than not, the researcher sees things as he has been trained—through the eyes of his mentors—rather than as the child watching the celebration of "The Emperor's New Clothes."[1] Creativity and innovativeness are related to seeing the old in new ways. Causality tends to be explained on the basis of old established "facts," the proof of which has not as yet been established (cf. Schechter[2]). John D. Benjamin[3] states,

> What is published is, almost of necessity, and with some important exceptions, seldom primary data themselves (the homologues of protocols of experiments in the experimental sciences), but anecdotally selected summaries of them, impressions about them, or secondary and tertiary inferences from them. . . . Thus, we find in fact that original theorizing in psychoanalysis, where it exists, is in general concerned with problems of clarification, of redefinition of accepted concepts and intervening variables in terms of logic and plausibility, in correcting one-sided points of view, or in introducing new explanatory concepts. Much *less often do we find the introduction of newly observed and described phenomena or relationships between phenomena, within the context of theoretical amplification or revision; and even more rarely the use of theory as a guide to observations and experiments aimed at testing its validity, generality, and predictive value* [italics mine]. . . . Where it is *not* possible, either directly or indirectly (as in the case of

intervening variables between two or more observables), either now or in the fore-seeable future through new psychological and biological method development, it is rather meaningless to speak of acceptance or rejection of theoretical proposi-tion except in a philosophic or esthetic sense. In any case, it seems necessary to dis-tinguish this sort of theorizing, at a great distance from clinical or experimental data although originally arising from it, from theory as we know it in science in general, with the constant two-way flow from observation and experiment to theory, and back again. [Cf. S. Arieti.[4]]

There have been three different clinical situations and one anecdotal experience in which the observations made, the operating paradigm, and the effective intervention have been different from, if not antithetical to, the usual and/or established models. In none of these have there been the discrete biochemical examinations as in the Mandell and Karno studies.

The symptoms and signs first delineated by Kanner[5] (noted by Karno) emphasize the withdrawal and noncommunicative aspects of the behavior of the child suffering from early infantile autism. In our own observations and in selecting similar per-ceptions of other authors, we felt the primary symptoms were related to an inability adequately to gate or filter external stimuli.[6] Whereas in this autistic child research we did some psychophysiological examinations, we did no serum or spinal fluid studies. In the study indicated these investigations would have vitiated the research design—*but there is no doubt that the definitive analyses would be those of the central nervous system catecholamines.* Our impressions included the avoidance of eye contact to keep from inconsistent, intolerable inputs whereas the self-stimulatory behavior was to cover, obliterate, or modulate unacceptable internal or external stimuli. (Cf., Hernandez-Peon et al.[7])

By placing these children in a perceptually isolated environment and grading the inputs, we were able to eliminate completely the self-stimulatory behavior, allow the development of contact with humans (partially related, we felt, to stimulus-action hunger[8]), teach the children to respond to directions, and, in some cases, teach them to meagerly use speech for communication. We currently have processed 5 children—all boys between 4 and 5 yr. of age—and our results are consistent with the response patterns eatablished during the perceptual isolation therapy and have been maintained in great part (up to 2 yr. after the experiment) with an ability to remain in contact with the environment. The emphasis in this model was on the importance of recognizing the defective *reizschutz* (protective shield)[9] and preparing an external environment to allow for adequate defense formation.

The second clinical experience[10] took place in an orthopedic hospital where we saw children who were placed in body casts or traction after being very physically active just before hospitalization. Boys suffering from Legg-Perthes disease (usually healthy, active 10-yr.-olds whose first symptom is that of pain in the hip or referred to the knee) are treated by immobilization with traction. Prior to placement in the trac-tion apparatus, the boys, although apprehensive about the hospitalization and separa-tion from home, were generally in a satisfactory mood except for the expected anxiety. However, once they were placed in traction and immobilized, all that was present was a severe, intractable, profound, and continuous depression. These children were unable to relate to the usually warm, friendly, and gentle staff. They did not eat, and sleep disturbances were universal. Contact with peers and schoolteachers was practically nonexistent and interest in the world about them could not be discerned.

On the hypothesis that depression represents aggression turned inward (not necessarily turned against a loved internalized object), boxing bags were hung from the traction apparatus, and the boys were given light boxing gloves and told to hit the bag as often and as hard as possible. Within 12 to 24 hr., all signs of depression had lifted, and the children were capable of positive interaction with the staff, including having energies available for academic learning. The emphasis in this model was on the importance of large-muscle discharge to the maintenance of psychic homeostasis (Cf. Mittelmann[11, 12] and Greenacre[13]).

The third clinical experience[14] dealt with a series of referrals of children having better-than-average intelligence, all of whom were failing in their schoolwork. It became evident that the mothers of these children suffered from maternal deprivation during their own childhood and, therefore, had no internal models upon whom to depend to administer proper maternal care to their own children, disaffecting them in a number of ways especially in their capacity to learn. Treatment was directed at giving the parents an opportunity to become dependent upon the therapist, develop a transitional object relationship, and then discard their usual emotional intuitive responses in favor of more satisfactory, gratifying, intellectually correct ones that met their own idiosyncratic needs and those of their family. Left to their own intuitive processes, they had failed miserably and continuously. Their responses were antagonistic to the proper helping of their children, and the emphasis in this instance was, in effect, "counterintuitive" based, in this model, on the concept that intuition is learned behavior. The correction that occurred included recognizing the inappropriate and inadequate object choices made in these mothers from the past and utilizing elements of learning theory to recorrect their psychopathology interrupting, thus, a cycle of maternal deprivation.

Within the last year, Dr. Jay Shurley,[15] professor of psychiatry at the University of Oklahoma Medical Center, returned from a visit to the Arctic Circle reporting the following anecdote. He and his colleagues observed that the children of the natives were effervescent and emotionally stable. These children went outside irrespective of the cold or darkness of the winters. This was in direct contrast to the children of the recent *émigrès* who not only remained housebound much of the year, but who had grave difficulties with large-muscle activities, and in whom depression was the pervasive affect. Most impressive and suggestive was that the depression even seemed to last beyond the time of their return to their homes in 1 of the southern 48 states. In each of these clinical examples, as with the concept of repetition compulsion, there needs to be an explanation beyond that of the metapsychological to that on a chemical, electrical, inter-, and intracellular level. The importance of feedback systems in which new stimuli are presented and new responses established cannot be dismissed as the possible base for the effectiveness of the psychotherapeutic process.

Finally, the naturalistic experiment of Powell et al.[16] must be noted. They found 11 children suffering from failure to thrive. As they examined the growth hormone in the serum of these youngsters, their presumptive diagnosis was that of panhypopituitarism. Since there was a shortage of pure extract of growth substance, the children were cared for by the regular nursery staff until the material could be obtained. Without any medication except normal feedings and the warmth, attention, and affection of superb nurses, the children began to grow and put on weight. Serum growth hormone studies revealed palpable amounts of this substance in the bloodstream. When the children approached the norm of the growth curve, they were discharged back to home, since foster homes were difficult to find. Reexamined after a period of time back home, they again had stopped growing or putting on weight, and concomitantly there was an absence again of the blood serum growth hormone. Therefore, the children were again ill, readmitted to the hospital, and given the same treatment as before. Obviously this treatment was the attention and care of concerned nurses without any hormonal therapy. The results were as expected. Again with the growth and development, there was a similar change in the functioning of the pituitary gland, clearly indicating the triggering mechanism of human contact for even normal biological processes. This serendipitous experiment closely reproduces in the psychosomatic arena the same scientific replicability required in following Koch's[17] bacteriological postulates.

Quod erat demonstrandum!

References

1. Anderson, H. C.: The emperor's new clothes." In: Lang, A. (Ed.): Yellow Fairy Book. New York, David McKay Co., 1962, pp. 27–32.
2. Schechter, M. D.: Psychiatric views and recommendations on orthopedic problems in children. Amer. J. Phys. Med. 41:231–233, 1962.
3. Benjamin, J. D.: Prediction and psychopathological theory. In: Jessner, L. and Pavenstedt, E. (Eds.): Dynamic Psychopathology in Childhood. New York, Grune & Stratton, 1959, pp. 6–77.
4. Arieti, S.: The present status of psychiatric theory. Amer. J. Psychiat. 124: 1630–1639, 1966.
5. Kanner, L.: Autistic disturbances of affective contact. Nerv. Child 2:217–250, 1943.
6. Schechter, M. D., Shurley, J. T., Sexauer, J. D., and Toussieng, P. W.: Perceptual isolation therapy: A new experimental approach in the treatment of children using infantile autistic defences. J. Amer. Acad. Child Psychiat. 8: 97–139, 1969.
7. Hernandez-Peon, R., Scherrer, H., and Jouvet, M.: Modification of electrical activity in cochlear nucleus during "attention" in unanesthetized cats. Science 123:331–332, 1956.
8. Lilly, J. C.: Mental effects of reductions of ordinary levels of stimuli on intact healthy persons. Psychiat. Res. Rep. Amer. Psychiat. Ass. 5:1–28, 1956.
9. Freud, S.: Beyond the pleasure principle. In: The Complete Psychological Works of Sigmund Freud, Vol. XVIII. London, Hogarth Press, 1955, pp. 7–64.
10. Schechter, M. D.: The orthopedically handicapped child. Arch. Gen. Psychiat. (Chicago) 4:247–253, 1961.
11. Mittelmann, B.: Motility in infants, children, and adults: Patterning and psychodynamics. Psychoanal. Stud. Child 9:142–177, 1954.
12. Mittelmann, B.: Motility in the therapy of children and adults. Psychoanal. Study Child 12:104–127, 1960.
13. Greenacre, P.: Infant reactions to restraint: Problems in the fate of infantile aggression. In: Trauma, Growth, and Personality. New York, W. W. Norton & Co. 1952, Chap. 3, pp. 83–105.
14. Schechter, M. D.: Bridge over troubled water—An interventive method in a cycle of maternal deprivation. J. Aust. New Zeal. Coll. Psychiat., 1971. To be published.

15. Shurley, J.: Personal communication, Nov. 18, 1971.
16. Powell, G. F., Brasel, J. A., Raite, S., and Blizzard, R. M.: Emotional depriva-tion and growth retardation simulating idiopathic hypopituitarism. New Engl. J. Med. 276:1279–1283, 1967.
17. Rosenau, M. J.: Koch's laws. As noted in: Preventive Medicine and Hygiene, 6th ed. New York, D. Appleton-Century Co., 1935, p. 645.

part 2
CHILDHOOD AND ADOLESCENCE

The Home in the Process of Learning

DANIEL M. LIPSHUTZ, M.D.

During a research project in a public school, my attention became focused upon a recurring observation: poor achievement, lack of concentration, and loss of drive and interest in the work and social activities in the classroom, leading to school failure, were important indicators of underlying emotional illness of various types and degree. Since the school's academic and administrative staffs were primarily trained as educators, lacking clinical insight, it soon became apparent that they were continuously missing the realistic origin of their problems with certain children and adolescents. Teachers and parents are primarily preoccupied with conduct and performance in the classroom. One could hardly expect them to consider other possibilities in the face of poor achievement. Thus, lack of interest, indolence, lethargy, daydreaming, absenteeism, truancy, as well as disobedience, aggressivity, hostility, and destructiveness to physical surroundings and to fellow classmates and teachers, were attributed to faulty curriculums and inadequate teachers.

At the weekly staff conferences, the principal and his assistants discussed the difficult children who were referred to them by the teachers for their consideration and disposition out of their classrooms because they

33

found it impossible to work with them. We learned that for years special teaching techniques and extra tutoring aids both within the school and at home were to no avail. Then, the method of distributing these children among the teachers considered more capable and efficient was thought might answer the recurring problems. But, since the underlying cause was not academic, the capable teachers were soon overloaded with difficult students, resulting in decreasing their efficiency and ego feelings. These teachers soon demanded that they be relieved of this, else they threatened to ask for transfer to other schools.

Research into the names of problem children presented at staff conferences in the preceding years indicated that almost all were still in evidence year after year, yet were still considered disciplinary and intellectual problems and treated as such. After many months of discussion and interpretation of the masking of real emotional illness by the manifestations of poor school achievement, the teaching staff gradually was able to grasp the underlying presence of physical and emotional illness, which gave real meaning to the label "the disturbed child."

A clinical study of each child's presenting symptoms together with his family history revealed that all principal entities of adult disturbance could be found among the disturbed children in this representative neighborhood school. Gould[1] showed that typical depression in children was disguised under surface behavior such as temper tantrums, boredom, restlessness, rebelliousness, hypochondriacal preoccupation, and vagrancy. Toolan[2] states that where depression is responsible for poor school achievement, a major complaint is difficulty of concentration. Hollon[3] has also observed that depression is the source of poor school achievement for certain children and adolescents. These observations take on special significance when it is realized that only rarely do teachers and parents associate these factors with school failure. They are practically never mentioned as reason for psychological evaluation.

Since it was definitely determined that changing of academic alternatives in no way influenced the process of learning in the disturbed child, we turned our attention to the home and the people in it who can alter the early development of these children, and the socioeconomic forces which played upon them. It is interesting to retrace the picture of the school and the area it served a generation ago, in comparison with its character and quality today. The neighborhood was formerly inhabited by an all-white, Jewish and Catholic, middle-class, comfortably established group of wage earners and small-business people. As a rule, they were actively interested in the education and activities of their children. The majority of these parents expected their offspring to do well scholastically and to progress to some form of higher education. They took active part personally and contributed to many community, religious, and secular agencies which dealt with the education and development of children. Thus, directly and indirectly, the parents played a part as a constant check on the educational agencies which created and administered the education of their children.

The parents equally stressed the same value of learning within the home and thought of it as a privilege to aid in the child's later competitive struggle in his business or professional life. With some parents, their drive for learning seemed inexhaustible. There were music and dancing lessons and Sunday school instruction interlaced with visits to the museum. The subtle form of introduction to learning was the general atmosphere created by books, discussions, and the tolerant guidance the parents offered in handling mystifying and confusing situations which came up in everyday life.

The great population movements created by the war and postwar industrial demands resulted in large immigrations of peoples from the West Indies, particularly from the island of Puerto Rico, and a large migration to the large manufacturing centers, primarily from the rural southern states. Because of their economic status, these newcomers replaced the middle-class whites who moved to new postwar dwellings or to the suburbs. In their concurrent competition for jobs, homes, and services, it was inevitable that both groups would eventually clash with harmful effects upon the community.

Because of the sudden and massive influx of both the black and Puerto Rican people into the community with little or no preparation for their coming by the city fathers, these parents were forced to fend for themselves, a task for which they were not fitted either emotionally or culturally. Trained neither educationally nor vocationally, the men were forced to accept minor, low-paying jobs which barely covered their daily needs for the family. In time, both parents were forced to seek employment in order to make ends meet. In homes in which one found a maternal or paternal grandmother, some semblance of a family unit was observed. In the others, the children often returned to empty houses, wandered about the streets, or were cared for temporarily by relatives and sympathetic neighbors. The more severely affected children, expecially among the blacks, were handicapped by the absence of the male parent either by desertion or because he had never become part of the household and had abandoned his responsibilities to the mother and to relief agencies.

Although the economic, social, and cultural factors were real and apparent, they triggered only the emotional regression in the parents which had already existed before their arrival in their country of adoption. Many of the disturbed children had come here at a school age already much beyond the period of the critical formative years, which would clearly indicate that the emotional deprivation in these children had taken place long before their arrival. It is, thus, unfair to attribute the failure of improving their intellectual capacity to the school system. Our study of the disturbed child in the classroom inevitably pointed to a relationship between the disturbance in the learning process and an emotional deprivation. We have often seen that with some disturbed children, a chance meeting with a naturally devoted and dedicated teacher results in evident improvement in the child's learning ability together with a change in the child's social and personal behavior. But we soon found that the improvement is only temporary if the teacher inadvertently withdraws her attention and warmth because of sudden demands made upon her by others in the classroom. The disturbed child soon returns to intense withdrawal, restlessness, rebelliousness, and asocial behavior accompanied by loss of interest, attention, and concentration.

Discussion

Present-day dynamic psychiatry has established that the formation of character and personality takes place in the first decade of life. The individual's drives which have molded these important functions have been strongly shaped and directed by his environment during that period. The most dominant person in the infant's growth and development in these formative years is the mother within the family unit.

From its inception, the embryo is dependent upon the mother physiologically to maintain its vital needs. The physical dependence upon her becomes progressively less important after birth, but the more complicated emotional growth to maturity continues throughout these critical years. During the first month of life, the infant remains comparatively an inert, passive mass, since the external sensory stimuli are still physiologically blocked so that "the great energy reservoir of the narcissistic phase"[4] can be completely replenished for the necessary aggressive functions which follow. Greenacre[5] spoke of the biological economy of birth so essential for the great energy demands following birth and during its process.

Spitz[6,7] and Ribble,[8] working independently, reported important observations on the then-unknown syndrome they had seen in large, well-organized pediatric services. Ribble called this illness, at the turn of the last century, "marasmus." Although careful physical examination and laboratory studies showed no pathological findings, the infants deteriorated steadily and had a high mortality. Incidental observation at that time seemed to point to insufficient stimulation both physically and emotionally of these children during their hospitalization, which Spitz later called "hospitalism."

Ribble[8] concluded that during development the child learns more sophisticated functions. Although the infant is still not prepared for an object relation in the first months of life, the mother is essential to the proper stimulation of the sucking reflex and chewing mechanism which will play a very important part in the development of speech and, later, in the creation of language. The bathing, drying, and fondling of the infant tend to stimulate groups of muscles of the chest cage and diaphragm, the auxillary mechanisms in the functions of breathing and speech.

Child psychoanalysts speak of the libidinization of the slowly developing sensory systems in the oral, acoustic, and optic areas, followed by the thermal and proprioceptive areas of movement, the anatomical pathways of which are helped to develop by proper stimuli. According to Spitz[7] the mother is necessary as a target against which the infant can direct its libidinal and aggressive drives. The growing number of stimuli returning to the afferent sensory systems by repetitive experiences with the mother helps the infant to individualize his own separate image. We may say that this is the first step in the formation of the ego or self—a primary, significant step in learning. As the infant's development continues and the child's emotional expressions of his drives provoke responses from the environment, these will, in turn, help to further strengthen these processes.

In their discussion of object relation, Hartmann, Kris, and Lowenstein[9] believe that the infant can form object relations only when there is "a collaborative action of the libidinal and aggressive drives." They believe that the infant directs its libidinal drives at an object labeled "good" and its aggressive drives at an object labeled "bad." The authors imply that this differentiation at this age indicates that perception has been accomplished and the percept delineated. Here, too, we have another giant step in the process of learning.

In the second half of the first year,[7] we see a progressive destructive activity appear. Hitting, biting, scratching, pulling, and kicking are used in the manipulative understanding of things, in order to learn about them and how to master them. The manipulation of things serve many purposes, primarily of perceptive orientation and of mastery. Here the mother serves as an object to be manipulated. In this way, the infant progressively begins his differentiation of self from the nonself. Soon there is an ability to differentiate animate from inanimate and, finally, between friend and stranger.

It is the mother's maternal warmth which will enhance or decrease the libidinal collaborative union with the instinctual aggressive drive. If the mother fails the child in this important function during the critical formative period, because of her own personality or character disturbance, or because of other unforeseen social or economic reasons, it will result in a variable reduction of the child's ability to bear frustration. Without this ability, it will become increasingly difficult to postpone satisfaction, so essential to normal emotional growth in a frustrating external world. Spitz[6] postulates that the infant must achieve the "reality principle" before any object perception can take place. It is only when the infant can accept the postponement of gratification that it will become free to direct its psychic energies to its environment and, thus, perceive the surrounding world from which it can learn; otherwise it remains narcissistically involved with itself and in an inner world of self-gratification.

Further growth and organization of the sensory-muscular system supply greater and more numerous outlets for the aggressive energies; with the aid of perception and thought, aggression is directed in the service of acquiring further mastery over objects in the environment as well as of obtaining skills, such as grasping and locomotion. This, in turn, widens the child's orientation in space, giving it more opportunity for discovery and new stimulation. The mother should be sufficiently stable at this period, so that she does not interfere with the child's budding adventures. If the child's increasing curiosity and mastery are beneficial to his emotional growth, they become more hazardous for the mother's precious possessions. She will be forced to manage her anxiety and postpone her gratification and pleasure until the child has reached a point in his development when he will be able to understand and accept commands. We can hardly blame the present-day mothers for their mounting anxiety, since our culture and civilization have produced objects in the child's environment which have become seriously dangerous for the child without constant supervision.

The earlier the emotional deprivation sets in, the greater are the noxious effects upon the child. The more the mother has helped the infant to separate from the "symbiotic orbit," as Mahler and her associates have shown[10]— that is, without undue strain upon his resources—the better equipped has the child become to "hatch" and to differentiate from the hitherto fused symbiotic object representations. Mahler and Furer[11] were especially impressed with the mutual selection of cues which infants present to indicate their needs. In a complex manner, the mother responds selectively to only certain of these cues. The infant alters his behavior in relation to these selective responses. He does so in a characteristic way: the resultant of his own innate endownment and the mother-child relationship. From this circular interaction emerge patterns of behavior that already show overall qualities of the child's personality. If the mother's mirroring function during infancy[10] is unpredictable, unstable, anxiety ridden, or hostile, if her confidence in herself as a mother is shaky, then the individuating child has to do without a reliable frame of reference for checking back, perceptually and emotionally, to the symbiotic partner.

Spitz[6] has observed that if the mother has been removed from the infant when the infant-mother relation has been good, the child shows a progressive mourning reaction if no adequate substitute is provided. The child begins to show greater restlessness, crying, and clinging to chance strangers. With further progression of the illness, apathy sets in. The presence of aggression in the normal child after 8 mo. of age, such as biting, hitting, and chewing, is conspicuously absent in the depressed child. If the mother is returned to the child after a limited period of depression, all functions seem to return in an exaggerated fashion. The aggression which he turned against himself is now directed outward, and the child begins to bite, scratch, and kick others instead of himself.

Comment

Although a percentage of teachers in the public schools themselves suffer from emotional disturbance, it is unfair to place the weight of blame upon the school system and its many sincere and dedicated teachers. Mumford[13] has shown that school authorities fear that the presence of a psychiatrist threatens the school's image. It is important to them to feel that their students "do not have those problems." The teacher-friends and the teacher-guides, he feels, believe that classroom performance is influenced by emotional and social factors. The authorities are at fault in persistently remaining suspicious of the professional services open to them. They are, at present, being forced to face the fact that sudden changes are upon them. They must recognize the difference that a disturbed child is not a disadvantaged child, and that both are not synonymous. In order to hide this unacceptable presence, they have adopted a new label, "the disruptive child."

An efficient use of the psychiatrist in the school, especially because of the limited number in the Child Guidance Bureau, is to localize his energies to the diagnosis of the disturbed child in the classroom, in order to separate him from the other children and place him in classrooms with specifically trained teachers. These teachers can, then, be prepared for what is to come. They can devote their time more efficiently to the children who can learn, instead of spending most of their time in the useless and frustrating effort of disciplining the disturbed child. This repeated situation has discouraged many excellent teachers, for they blame themselves for the failure of their pupils.

References

1. Gould, R. E.: Suicide problems in children and adolescents. Amer. J. Psychother. 19:228, 1965.
2. Toolan, J. M.: Depression in children and adolescents. Amer. J. Orthopsychiat. 32:404, 1962.
3. Hollon, T. H.: Poor school performance as a symptom of masked depression, in children and adolescents. Amer. J. Psychother. 25:258, 1970.
4. Klein, M.: Envy and Gratitude. New York, Basic Books, 1957.
5. Greenacre, P.: The biological economy of birth. Psychoanal. Stud. Child 1:31, 1945.
6. Spitz, R.: Hospitalism: An inquiry into the genesis of psychiatric conditions in early childhood. Psychoanal. Stud. Child 1:53, 1945.
7. Spitz, R.: Aggression: Its Role in the Establishment of Object Relations: Drives, Affects, Behavior. New York, International Universities Press., 1953.
8. Ribble, M.: The Rights of the Infant. New York, Columbia University Press, 1945.
9. Hartmann, H., Kris, E., and Lowenstein, R. M.: Notes of the theory of aggression. Psychoanal. Stud. Child 3:12, 1949.
10. Mahler, M. S., with Furer, M.: On Human Symbiosis and the Viscissitudes of of Individuation. Vol. 1, Infantile Psychosis. New York, International Universities Press, 1968.
11. Mahler, M. S., and Furer, M.: Certain aspects of the separation: Individuation phase. Psychoanal. Quart. 32:1–14, 1963.
12. Spiegel, L. A.: The self, the sense of self, and perception. Psychoanal. Stud. Child 14:81–109, 1959.
13. Mumford, E.: Teachers' response to school mental health programs. Amer. J. Psychiat. 125:75–81, 1968.

Discussion by Ursula M. von Eckardt, Ph.D.

I agree with Dr. Lipshutz that disturbance in learning is a consequence of behavior disturbances such as aggressiveness, lethargy, passivity, and disinterest; and that this is related to the culture shock experienced by children of migrants, particularly Puerto Ricans who have moved from the island to New York or Negroes from rural areas or small towns in the deep South, and to the emotional atmosphere in the homes of these children. It is also quite true that the average schoolteacher, particularly the white, middle-class urban teacher is ill equipped by training, by her own cultural conditioning, and by the context in which she is forced to operate to understand and cope with the complex psychosocial factors which influence the manner in which her pupils—I won't say "learn" because she seldom has any way of finding out what they actually learn—perform the rituals through which the pupils are rewarded or accepted in the system.

If now "mental illness" is introduced as a causative factor to explain the poor performance of the problem child, all the categories and presuppositions with which the teacher operates are threatened. Indeed, I would go further and assert that any teacher willing to accept, not Dr. Lipshutz' empirical observations because even educators can see these now, but his theoretical framework and basic assumptions, could not long survive in our school system.

The explanations of the specific behavior Dr. Lipshutz observed, however, does not necessarily require any "in-depth" analysis of mother-child relationship or any determination of mental illness. Take, for example, the case of the 12-yr.-old Puerto Rican boy who continually came to school several hours late and made trouble by forcing a girl from her seat, claiming it was his. I learned, to my teutonic obsessional dismay, that in Puerto Rican culture nothing, absolutely nothing, starts on time. Today, in 1972, certain activities do start within an hour of the announced starting time, but a school, particularly a poor school for lower-class children who are not expected to have clocks or watches at home, begins more or less sometime in the morning and ends when everybody feels he has had enough. I am not exaggerating much. But it would be, I believe, committing what I am going to call the psycho-analytical fallacy to assume that people from a Latin culture who habitually come late for everything are therefore, let's say, unconsciously hostile. What they really are is, quite consciously, indifferent to the value of time.

Nor are Latin classrooms very formal affairs. There are places where everybody wanders in and out (in rural schools this includes goats and chickens or the babies that must be guarded while the older children study). Surely the New York City schoolroom is a strange sort of prison-like place by comparison. That the boy should challenge the girl is equally proper among *machos*. If there are not enough chairs to go around, it is the natural order of things in any Latin lower-class environment, and, I suspect, in American Negro culture as well, that the boys sit and the girls stand. In this particular case, apparently the boy was ill—or so Dr. Lipshutz' additional reports indicate—but I would warn that without a very careful study of all the socio-cultural factors which mold and shape human behavior it is as misleading to label conduct "hostile," "ill," "aggressive," etc., as it is to label it "inmoral," "lazy," or "delinquent."

Dr. Lipshutz points out some of these factors himself. It is certainly correct that Puerto Rican migrant families (not immigrant, please: this is part of the picture, they wish predominantly to return home and never quite abandon or emotionally break with their own island) are too concerned with immediate material needs to worry very much about whether the children attend school or not. Moreover, although the upper layer of the Puerto Rican lower class, which makes up most migrants who must have enough initiative to move from the rural zone to San Juan, and from San Juan to Florida or New Jersey and then to New York City, are highly socially mobile and often attach great importance to education in the abstract; however, they do not realize that daily school attendance as such is important.

Minor illness, needing the child to run errands, the absence of a pair of shoes, simply the unwillingness of the child to go—all these are considered adequate reasons for not sending him.

The absence of men is also a correct observation, although I doubt that their presence would change the children's truancy pattern or interest in school. Mother and grandmother run the house and the children, anyway.

A great many other, more general cultural factors and values are involved which—without any reference whatsoever to psychopathology or emotional disturbance of any kind—tend to explain why Puerto Rican children in particular, and Latin and southern Negro children as well, fail to adapt and learn in a modern urban WASP school. Among these are the Latin negative value of competition, the higher value placed on "friendliness" than on "intelligence," the child centeredness which cannot understand or apply rules (the child is like an animal to be tolerated or ignored as long as possible and then kicked or physically removed when he becomes irritating), and the very high level of noise and the chronic malnutrition which make for a high rate (one estimate says 31.6 percent among Puerto Rican adults) of mental retardation. One should also mention the obvious: the language barrier.

I have nothing much to say about Dr. Lipshutz' "discussion," which seems to me a fairly straightforward presentation of psychoanalytical child development theory. But I do believe that there is quite a leap, over an unchartered territory of logical and hypothetical connections, to the empirical observations made in the beginning of the paper. I do not think it is necessary to speculate about the deprivation of mother love or pathological conditions during infancy in order to explain what can be fairly simply explained in socioanthropological terms.

I agree with Dr. Lipshutz that it is "unfair" to blame "sincere and dedicated teachers"—indeed, I would like to get away from the notion of *blaming* anybody for anything—but it is nevertheless quite easily demonstrable that the character of our competitive, middle-class-oriented schools and schoolteachers and the values in terms of which "learning" is determined and rewarded present insurmountable culture shocks to the Spanish-Latin and rural American lower-class Negro child, and that the response to the shock is a kind of behavior which is interpreted by the WASP educators as school failure. But overpsychologizing the problem is, in my opinion, as misguided as dealing with it exclusively in traditional educationist terms.

And now that I have dispatched Dr. Lipshutz, let me make some comments of my own. These are based on the study of Puerto Rican middle-class, socioculturally advantaged adolescents in the context of their own culture.

Of course, the home is important—not only in the process of learning but also in the process of school success, which is something else again. The family dynamics and the interplay of personalities in the home set the patterns of the human relationship within which the growing young person is able to cope. We have found, in questioning high school students about their "favorite" teachers and subjects and about their abilities and performance record, that the students "learned most" and "studied hardest" with those teachers who most closely resembled the personality profiles of their own fathers, mothers, or other significant persons. Those with highly authoritarian and aloof fathers preferred and learned most from authoritarian and aloof male teachers; those with warm, loving and egalitarian parents preferred and learned most from the warm, loving, egalitarian teachers, etc. This was irrespective of their abstract preference for an "authoritarian" or "egalitarian" teacher.

Clearly, learning—at least school learning—is always mediated by an interpersonal relationship and the least anxiety-arousing one: the personality type that is familiar and hence predictable is the most productive.

Perhaps girls pose fewer learning problems in school because most schoolteachers are women; at least some serious investigations should be made to determine if Negroes learn more from Negro teachers, and so on. Evidence is mounting that children perform best on intelligence tests when these are administered by persons of their own ethnic group, under familiar conditions. What applies here to personality type might surely apply to cultural types as well.

To the degree to which school performance is stressed at home, to that extent is it utilized by the youngster as an instrument for manipulating parents or significant persons. A boy who hates or resents his father, will punish the latter by "failing" his classes. This is particularly the case in a culture such as the Puerto Rican where direct, openly expressed hostility is taboo. A traditionally raised Puerto Rican boy who does not want to study, say, accounting, when his father insists on it, would never dare to defy the father openly. But he would consistently fail all classes remotely related to this subject until the father abandoned this career choice for the boy. Conversely, we have observed that a parent, particularly a father, may engage in active rivalry with his son, overtly urging the boy to study and get good grades, but convertly doing everything possible (e.g., turning up the radio "real loud" when the boy has to concentrate on homework, failing to provide study space, interrupting constantly) to cause the boy to fail. Usually such fathers were formally uneducated and felt inferior to their high school-or college-attending sons.

The student who wants approval at home and earns it through good grades will seek to obtain these grades—very often through cheating. The parents get what they ask for, and if these are A's on the report card, that is what they will get, no matter how they have to be obtained. Ambitious B+ students outcheat the D students who are uninterested in grades.

Many other factors and specifics could be listed, varying somewhat with age, culture, attitude, personality, etc. But certainly home and school are merely two parts of the growing youngster's life and the events in one most assuredly affect the behavior in the other. In the same way, emotional states, like physical ones, affect input and outcome on the level of reasoning. Intelligence and learning are far more complex still and are affected intricately by disposition, circumstance, conditioning, inclination, emotion—the list of factors is virtually infinite—that it is no longer possible to deal adequately with anything else than the total ecology of the human situation, in school as well as elsewhere.

What we need, therefore, are intensive studies which deal specifically and in detail with the whole long catalog of psychological, social, and anthropological factors involved in learning and schooling. And, perhaps, a clearer insight into our own assumptions, values, and biases which we apply not only to the school system but to all our institutions in such a manner that we judge all who do not fit, adapt, or adjust either as failures to be morally rejected or as "mentally ill" to be perhaps less harshly dismissed, but nevertheless to be thoroughly misunderstood.

The Gamines

JOSE GUTIERREZ*

It was only through a frankly personal commitment that I was enabled to study the lives of that strange group of children who form a type of miniature guerilla band at large in the urban areas of Colombia, labeled depreciatively by the Colombian populace "the gamines." To induce a feeling for the word as it is generally spoken, the reader might try pronouncing it with a tone of voice combining fear and disgust, uneasiness and weary fatalism generally reserved for natural disasters, much as in medieval times one might have said "the plague."

The subject

The gamines are children of the streets. They constitute a permanent, self-contained, and rather highly structured social group, particularly in Bogota where their number may be estimated at between 2000 and 5000. A gamine often begins his life in the streets at the age of 4 or 5 and from that

*This investigation has been supported by a five-year grant from the Foundations' Fund of Research in Psychiatry.

time until he is perhaps 15 he ranges with freedom through the city, playing, fighting, begging, stealing, working occasionally at odd jobs, and amusing himself at the expense of adult dignity. A mixture of teasing, joking, and grotesque but vibrant humor seasons all of his behavior, particularly when his path is thwarted by any institution, ritual, or constriction. He runs rampant through the streets of Bogota, be they those in the center of town or those in the most elegant residential areas, thrusting his ragged, clownlike little figure on the unwilling consciousness of the adult world and showing it that its opinion is to him only a source of amusement.

Since all ties with his family are broken, generally irrevocably, the street provides not only the gamine's stage for exhuberant theatrics and source of survival, but his place of rest as well. He sleeps beneath the cover of newspapers or funeral announcements, cocooned with his partner or a few friends in the rubble of a construction site, beneath a parked car, or simply on the sidewalk, bundled against the wall of a building. Sleep, like everything else in his life, is unpredictable, subject to circumstances and dependent on his ability to adapt. Often awakened by the damp cold of early morning in Bogota, he will take advantage of the afternoon sun and warm pavement, sprawling haphazardly with his friends, lying like war-broken bodies, in the midst of the rush hour, taking his chances with the misstep of a pedestrian or the prodding of the police.

When he awakens, he has no precise plan and begins to wander, generally directed by hunger, but uncertain as to how the need can be satisfied and sure only that it will depend on his own cleverness in taking advantage of whatever situation presents itself to him. If he encounters a man getting out of his car, he will ask if he can watch it for a peso, but if he happens along while the man is getting into his car, he will demand the same for already having watched it. He is not a beggar by nature but is perfectly willing to beg and is adept at it as well. If he judges that a woman will respond through pity, he is soft voiced, humble, and the archetype of abject misery. If he judges that one man is bored with the whining of beggars and will respond only to directness, his gaze is steady and his voice strong, or another through confusion or embarrassment, he will adopt a threatening and aggressive approach. His judgment is seldom mistaken. Similarly, although he does not live by theft and has neither use nor concern for acquisition, he is often willing, out of either the necessity of hunger or the emotional necessity of a dare, to steal food, hubcaps, windshield wipers, or whatever unattended objects present themselves.

His day is filled with improvisations, incidents, surprises, opportunities, hopes, risks, threats, and escapes. His relationships with others like himself, which form a central part of his life, share the same uncertain and constantly shifting quality. They meet together to share spoils (either by wish or by force), exchange goods, form working teams, roughhouse, and amuse themselves, but beneath all of this activity is a constant search for an emotional support which is elusive and impossible to predict from one day to the next.

The approach

If the reader has had experience with the methods of sociological investigation, he will recognize this early that the gamines provided, at best, a difficult subject for such a study as this. Among the obvious methodological problems which I faced in approaching these children was that of understanding and defining their actions and attitudes, while avoiding the imposition of conventional social values and eliminating preconceived and culturally biased concepts and terminology first from my own mind and thence from my study. It was partially for this reason that I chose a psychoanalytical approach in my investigation of the gamines.

I held the belief that facing the question of gaminism, without preliminary definitions or prejudicial categorization, was strictly in line with the spirit of psychoanalysis. The wide scope which Freud succeeded in encompassing within his method should make it applicable to any social study dealing with ways of life differing from the usual. Unfortunately, however, present psychiatric practice has developed methodological patterns which have limited its potential in this direction.

Those of us who have worked with patients coming to our offices in search of help (that is to say in the habitual psychoanalytic manner) have the tendency to classify life styles under the categories of healthy or neurotic, rational or irrational. It is difficult for us to part with the idea that the more an individual takes advantage of the resources offered him by society, the better off both he and society will be. There are, there have been, and there will probably continue to be people aware of their conflicts, disturbed by them, and prepared to ask for help.

This was obviously far from the case with the gamines, however, who are notorious for making any adult who attempts to interfere with or to alter their way of life a victim of their hostility and ridicule. Tossing about observations concerning culture and society, armed with the libido theory, with a couch or without one, I could not begin to understand these gamines, so radically different from the patients who willingly looked to me for help. I would have been lost from the beginning if I had attempted to work with these devilish children with the idea of unilaterally molding them to conventional attitudes of life patterns.

I believed that one of the causes of failure in the previous attempts to approach the gamines had been that their adult "benefactors" had displayed an obstinate and blinding need to convince them in earnest tones of the extremity of their social deviance and show them "the error of their ways" as a first step toward "civilizing" them. The result was a symbiotic relationship in which the adults were able to satisfy their crusading zeal on the pagans, while the pagans willingly profited from whatever material benefits were offered. Of course, with depressing predictability the adults were frustrated by an incapacity to effect any genuine change, while the gamines endured another in a series of relationships in which they were forced to express defensive pride at the expense of developing a desired emotional faith.

The poor results produced by these initial attempts had their origins in a lack of precise knowledge of the psychological and sociological characteristics of the problem, particularly in a mistaken conception of the psychological dynamics of the benefactor-gamine relationship. Objective investigation was therefore necessary: effective altruism is not possible without a clear understanding of the motives of both parties. Although such an objective investigation in which the subject of the study becomes an object appears potentially contradictory to aid in human development, psychiatry has made them compatible through its particular combination of human knowledge and curative stimulation.

The basic characteristic of psychoanalysis, which differentiates it from such studies as sociology or anthropology, is that its aim should never cease to be curative, to provide the subject with an insight into possibilities which were before excluded to him and enable him to choose freely from among these rather than being directed by compulsion. Only with this purpose clearly in mind may its process by analytic. Therefore, psychoanalysis does not deal with human beings as static facts or objects, but rather interests itself in human potentials and the dynamics of development, directly affecting this development through the personal relationship between analyst and patient, a relationship which is completely lacking between investigator and object.

Thus I decided on a psychoanalytic approach, but not that of a traditional analyst who waits in his office for patients to come to him. I could not capture gamines and tie them to the couch. If I wanted to become a part of their lives, I would not only have to go out into the streets with them but also have to do without many of the other formal props, mental, methodological, and physical, which define and limit traditional psychoanalytic practices.

The psychoanalytic relationship

I had established that both the nature of the gamines and my own aims required an approach which was personal and psychoanalytic, rather than factual and statistical. But the central question remained as before, "What type of relationship could be effective both from a curative and from an investigational point of view and how were its first steps to be implemented?" The constant turmoil of the gamines' lives defies both prediction and restriction. Therefore, any approach to them must be fluid and develop largely by innovation rather than by plan.

Representative of the erratic behavior which posed my problem is their favorite pastime *"lincharse,"* in which groups of 2 or 3 children will catch rides on the backs of buses or cars, often during rush-hour traffic in Bogota. This is done with no particular destination in mind; it is a game, pure exhilaration, and the ride lasts until the vehicle stops, they fall, a policeman forces them off, or (best of all) an irate driver stops and gives futile chase. If the gamines behaved in this way, one could not hope, even if he wishes, to calm them down, gather them in a fixed place at a fixed time, and, according to a well-defined plan, give them routine tests and psychological examinations. At least one could not impose this type of unfamiliar discipline on them without destroying the freedom of action which is the supposed basis of psychoanalysis.

On the other hand, it was impossible to imagine that to gain my ends I would have to learn to hitch rides on the backs of buses or completely displace myself into the other uncertainties of gamine life. This state of absolute personal uncertainty is a tyrranical demand with which science is basically incompatible. My only hope was that they would hitch on to my investigation into gaminism and, through this voluntary interest on their part, I would really be able to know and share their lives.

Psychoanalysis demands a relationship whereby the psychoanalyst becomes involved in the vicissitudes of the patient's life without necessarily becoming a permanent part of his world. Sociologically, this psychoanalytic participation implies a social function which is not a permanent element in the life of the one who is being psychoanalyzed. Freud described it as a substitution which is meant to be transitory. Just as with children parents alter their role at each stage of development, so it is with psychoanalysis. The analyst's substitutive role should change naturally as the patient achieves the growth necessary for him to attain a greater vision of alternatives and the ability to choose among them, and finally, the psychoanalytic relationship becomes a thing of the past.

Unfortunately, however, psychoanalysis has been corrupted by many who practice it in that they have developed excessively rigid patterns for this substitutive function. Lacking faith in the subtle spirit of Freud's idea, they have dogmatized his technique. The result has been that they have stripped the substitutive process of its natural and fluid quality and taken from it all the flavor of a first-hand human experience. They have succeeded only in depriving themselves of their own spontaneity, in transforming themselves into tools for "working on" their patients and transforming their patients into objects of the psychoanalytic technique.

It was, therefore, fortunate that my psychoanalytic relationship with the gamines was impossible to program, and I was forced to rely on spontaneity and immediate personal judgment, for had rigid planning been possible, I would perhaps have fallen into the same routine which for many years I had wanted to alter. Worse yet, if I had used dogmatic techniques, I would have been vulnerable to the suspicion of the gamines who, with their own spontaneous freedom of expression, are expert in the testing and exposure of poses.

First contact

As it turned out, my wife and I were, without relying on a previously devised scheme but through a natural series of events, able to effect the psychoanalytic substitution by partially replacing the *galladas* (gangs) with a new social system in which we figured centrally. Through the resulting relationship, we were able not only to participate in the gamines' lives and to gain their confidence, but also to coexist without crucial alterations in our own life style. The truth is that I had not encouraged the gamines to form a "gang" with me and my family, but the circumstances of having made friends with a couple of gamines led to precisely that: "the doctor's gang."

In order to explain how this came about, it is necessary to describe the original structure of gamine society. The gangs, or *galladas* as they call themselves, are groups of 6 to 12 children, dominated by a leader, known as a *largo* or *perro* (dog), which "holds" a certain well-defined territory. There are three principle cohesive forces binding these children to the *gallada*. The first is an exterior force consisting of police persecution, adult hostility, and aggression by other groups. The second is the force exerted by the *largo*, which is a peculiar combination of protectiveness, domination, and exploitation. The third cohesive force consists of ties between pairs of individuals within the *gallada*. In reality, it is these pairs which make up the *gallada*. The closeness of the pairs vacillates constantly between casual friendship and intense mutual dependence. Having a friend of this latter type is known as having a *"vale"* (voucher) or *"iman"* (magnet). It may be either a relationship of equals or, more commonly, a domination-submission relationship in which one protects the other and the second admires and fears the first. Whatever its dynamics, it provides each individual not only with support and aid in the violation of norms, laws, and moral customs, but, most important, with an emotional attachment to fill the void left by the absence of family.

As it happened, we were in contact with two *vales,* Alvaro Perez and Juan Gonzales, whose former relationship with some of the members of our team encouraged at least the necessary initial, wary belief in the honesty of our intentions. These two *vales* gradually appeared more frequently at our office and, finally, as will later be seen, came to live with my family and me in our house. Without the emotional closeness and bizarre loyalty of Gonzales and Perez to myself and my family, we could not have accomplished any type of substitution for the closed and *largo*-dominated *galladas* of the gamines. As it were, however, under the influence of this original pair, a *gallada* slowly crystallized among those children whom we had chosen for the study, in the dynamics of which we played a central part.

Gamines and nongamines

In the beginning phases of our contact with the gamines, while "the doctor's gang" was in the process of formation, our primary problem was in developing in the children a faith in ourselves and our intentions, which were entirely alien to their previous experience. It was an infinitely slow mental adjustment on both sides. We had, after all, been blind to them for most of our lives, carefully avoiding noticing them or feeling their needs, isolating ourselves from them, as all of the citizens of Colombia do as efficiently as possible. They, in turn, had for the most part received nothing but brutal treatment or indifference from adults and had accordingly calloused themselves effectively by turning the pain and rejection received into profound distrust, arrogance, and ridicule. The changes which had to take place could not be forced; they had to develop naturally and voluntarily.

There was also, however, a second problem facing us at all times. This one was methodological and centered around the question of what individuals we should work with and what specific criteria were to be used in their selection. The following conversation with Gonzales about the relationship between adults and the gamines shed light for us on both these problems:

"The gamines are enemies of the rich," said Gonzales.

"All gamines?" I asked.

"No, not all of them. There are the "*chupagruesos*" [toadies, those who suck up to someone, those who curry favor]." Here, Gonzales made a descriptive mimic, impossible to translate into words—a mixture of genuflexions, sly looks with lips puckered up as if sucking on something—and said, "Please, sir, would you give me a peso if I watch your car?"

"We fight them and call them stool pigeons," continued Gonzales in order to explain the contempt which is evoked by the whiny slyness of these submissive children. "Then they get mad, and when they see us taking care of somebody's car, they'll say, 'Ay, so you're a *chupagrueso, too.*' And you answer, 'Me, a *chupagrueso*? I don't suck up to anybody so he'll give me money, clothes, food, anything.'" And now Gonzales' face and gestures have become tough, very much like a cowboy in a Western.

The difference between the gamines and the *chupagruesos* rest on two clean and simple norms: the gamines take pleasure in showing arrogance toward adults and have an undisguised hatred of the rich, both of which are lacking in the *chupagruesos*. Those who do not display these forms of bravado are aliens to the society of the gamines, become the butt of their mockery and disdain, and are forced to remain in a limbo between the worlds of the *galladas* and that of conventional society.

"The *chupagruesos* sell out. They are rats. Even when they live in the streets like we do, they are rats. They are bootlickers and do not live in *galladas* the way we do because they have squealed on others from time to time. They are afraid that somebody will roll them to take revenge. If they are not taken care of by their families or some institution, they have contracts—assured daily charity from a home, restaurant, or shop."

This description made by Gonzales suggests the conclusion that to be a true gamine one has to show a determined and consistent antagonism toward adults. If a child is not, in gamine terminology, "*firme*" (unbending), he does not belong to the closed society of the gamine.

At this point, however, I must introduce an apparent contradiction. The gamines also have "contracts." Nevertheless, in this, as in all relationships with adults, they do not surrender their independence. The "contracts" which they have are entirely unilateral; they do not imply any commitment on the part of the child, at least in his own mind. They are deceptive "agreements" which the child enters into and breaks with pleasure. The contract can last only as long as the benefactor's patience holds out.

Gonzales gave an example of this type of relationship when he asked a well-dressed young man in the street for a cigarette in his habitually aggressive manner. The young man at first refused, but then, thinking better of the possible consequences, turned and said, "I'll give you one if you watch my car." After Gonzales had accepted the cigarette, one of the psychiatrists in our team jokingly suggested that he had behaved like a *chupagrueso*. Gonzales clarified the situation by saying, "In the first place, he was the one who offered me the job; I only accepted the cigarette. And in the second place, who's going to watch his car if I'm already leaving?"

In this incident we see one example of a pattern of behavior followed by the gamines with incorruptible consistency in order to maintain their independence. The combination of arrogance and detachment and the constant defiance and ridicule to which they subject adults is founded in a general disregard for conventional manners and morals which begins at a very early age. This antagonism dictates for them implicit codes of behavior which are a powerful factor in consolidating their peculiarly hermetic society, replete with its own customs, language, and values.

A new dimension for the study

Initially, my plan had been a study in depth of 20 gamines. I later changed this plan, however, because I was struck with a new idea. I was strongly interested in the fact that there existed children whose lives seemed to be influenced by environmental and social conditions quite similar to those of the gamines but whose characters, values, and way of life were in fact very different. This observation suggested that the causes or origins of gaminism did not lie so much in environmental determinism as most people would have expected.

In order to test this observation and take the study into a more purely psychological realm, in which for me its primary value lay, two steps were necessary. The first was to clarify our definition of gaminism and, using this as a criterion, select those individuals who represented its purest strain. This selection was done by both objective and subjective means. Besides establishing our own criteria, in which the basic elements were alienation and rebellion against conventional social practices and values, we devised and administered questionnaires to take a representative sampling of society's definition of gaminism. Using these combined criteria, we chose 10 individuals from among those with whom contact had been made.

The second step was to match with each of these 10 a child who had experienced similar social and environmental circumstances, but was not a gamine. Thus if, for instance, we had selected a gamine whose family had been affected by the Colombian political violence (*ha violencia*) or had an alcoholic father, we chose a nongamine whose family was similarly affected, and so on with each characteristic. It was, of course, difficult to correlate several variables simultaneously but we were eventually successful to a good degree, as can be seen in Table 1, which provides statistics on the social backgrounds of the 20 children (10 gamines and 10 nongamines) whom we eventually selected, together with their most notable characteristics.

With the selection process completed, we could say that the core of the study was actually underway. The attempt to understand each life in its own uniqueness, to find the causes for the direction it had taken, and hopefully also to bring the individual to a recognition of those causes and offer him the power to choose alternatives, these were tasks which now faced us.

Toward a renewal in psychoanalysis

Owing to the previously described flexible and personal psychoanalytic approach to the study which followed, one can perhaps imagine the complex shifting of roles, statuses, and values which resulted both for the children and for ourselves. For all of us who participated in this work these interchanges were vital experiences, awakening new emotions, opening new horizons, new possibilities, new freedom, and this is precisely where its psychoanalytic value lay.

For many years the Colombian government, voluntary associations, and many civic-minded individuals had worked at trying to solve the "plague of gaminism." None, however, had been even minimally successful. It was, and is, my belief that the primary cause of these failures lay in the fact that the individuals involved had been unwilling to submit themselves to any fluid interchange of roles, retaining and defending instead the static and irreconcilable positions of benefactor and social bankrupt, Christian and urban savage. Therefore, the social and emotional abyss which separated the life of the gamine from the life of those who desired to "improve" him remained unbridged, as profound and impossible as before. Their sole object had been the conversion of these children into respectable members of Colombian society; they desired sincerely, in fact felt a psychological need, to help these children, but were paralyzed by their own conventional attitudes which prohibited any valid communication or transmission of experience or values between the two groups. This was precisely the approach which I was attempting to avoid.

As a result of having undergone a rigorous psychoanalysis myself, I had been able to free myself of the "need to convert" and did not experience the "psychological dependence" which had been a mote in the eye of my predecessors. On the other hand, I could feel, in part, the stigma of being a gamine. Through my intimate relations with them I could appreciate the pain of social ostracism, of police persecution, and of the rejection they faced because of their appearance. A notable example of the causes for my empathy occurred when our landlord suggested, in a diplomatic manner typical of Bogotanos, that we move from our combination residence and office. His reasons were that the building had become undesirable since a pack of ragged, dirty children had begun to frequent it.

Aside from my personal experience, I was also able to determine the attitudes of Colombian society toward the gamines by traditional sociological measurements. This was done by means of two questionnaires given to a stratified and representative sampling of the population of Bogota— the first intended to determine the qualifications established for gaminism and the second, more statistically sophisticated, aimed at determining social attitudes toward these children.

Briefly, the results of these two samples indicate that (a) gamines are generally defined as rebellious children without firm family ties, associated in gangs which form a defined social group opposed to adult society, and (b) gamines are feared and rejected by children and the poor to whom they represent the most immediate threat, are looked upon with indifference by the upper class, and are habitually regarded by all as an example of the irresponsibility of the state and not as a personal concern. The questionnaires also disclosed that those who held the most firmly authoritarian concept of family structure and those with the greatest aspirations toward upward mobility were strongest in their rejection of the gamines.

These sociological findings were perfectly in accord with my psychoanalytic experience with the gamines: I felt myself at times, through association with them, stigmatized, pessimistic, and abandoned and could share with these children their rebellious, violent, and hopeless world.

This correlation between personal psychoanalytic experience and sociological data produced for me a surprising revelation. I had been looking for a rigorous sociological methodology to supplement my limited personal experience with the gamines, but discovered that the psychoanalytical approach, individualistic and utilizing subjective personal involvement, had already established a truth to which the complex statistical investigations were only a supporting footnote.

This discovery, however, should not have been so surprising if we had taken into account the broad social implications of Freud's original ideas. In combining both investigative and curative elements Freud created between the analyst and patient an essentially new type of social relationship, quite different in its dynamics from any of those which the patient has experienced in normal social life. The investigative or analytical element contributes to maintaining a distance between patient and psychiatrist which is critical for mutual objectivity and a necessary degree of independence for each. On the other hand, the dynamic curative or developmental element stimulates emotional involvement, evolves deeply personal responses, and strengthens the human solidarity of the two.

Through this combination of elements a relationship encouraging freedom and objectivity, confidence, respect, and support is developed which differs radically from the patterns of competition, dependence, and restraint which seem to characterize conventional social relationships.

Thus the psychiatrist plays a critical, though transitory, role in the actual life of the patient, the purpose of which is to enable and encourage the latter to develop two concurrent abilities. First the therapist participates in the life of the patient under special conditions as an investigator who is not an intruder extracting information for later use, but rather a mirror which serves to develop in the patient his capacity to observe himself. As soon as this capacity for self-observation is developed, the patient continues his own psychoanalysis. He becomes the object of his own investigative reasoning and the subject of his own therapeutic practice. To put this in other terms, the psychoanalytic process reaches a point at which the analyst may be present or absent, but his function has begun to transfer itself to the patient, who ultimately must continue independently of him.

Second, the analyst's relationship with the patient allows the latter to develop a new faith in himself and others, a fresh sense of the potential inherent in other human relationships, and emotional confidence to transfer this example to the world at large, thus fulfilling the new potential which he sees.

Unfortunately, however, the hermetic atmosphere of the consultation room too often defines the boundaries of both the patient's new insight into himself and of the ability to form the new type of relationship, making transferral of either to his external social context difficult at best. Patient and analyst, once out of the room, are again absorbed into the system which was the original cause of the difficulty, and psychoanalysis has become merely another social anesthetic, providing temporary relief for the pain and confusion which the patient feels in his "other world" or perhaps simply enabling him to endure that pain more gracefully.

In recent years much has been said about the socialization of psychoanalysis. Diverse means have been employed in an attempt to refresh the rarified atmosphere of the musty couches and sealed consultation rooms.

But group therapy, psychodrama, therapeutic communities, community psychiatry, environmental therapy, sensitivity training, group encounter, behavioral therapy, and other methods have done little either to liberate the patient-analyst relationship from its traditional confining context or to spread the application of Freud's principles to society as a whole.

The experience of having gone out into the streets with the gamines and of having had them become a part of the life of my family, the gratifying results of having established in my practice a freer and more spontaneous approach, less circumscribed by dogmatic theoretical procedures, and the deep response and honest interchange which these evolved in these difficult children have convinced me that if psychoanalysis is willing to take on the responsibility of a free and open confrontation with problems like gaminism it will in the future make profound contributions to social change and thus fulfill the complete potential inherent in Freud's legacy.

Table 1. A Comparison of 10 Gamines and 10 Nongamines

Characteristics	Number of Gamines	Number of Nongamines
10 yr. old	—	2
11 yr. old	1	—
12 yr. old	2	4
13 yr. old	5	4
Estimated age 10–13	1	—
14 yr. old	1	—
Total	10	10
Rural father	6	4
Urban father	3	4
Unknown father	1	2
Total	10	10
Urban mother	4	3
Rural mother	6	7
Total	10	10
Father living	9	8
Father unknown	1	2
Total	10	10

Table 1 (Continued).

Characteristics	Number of Gamines	Number of Nongamines
Mother living	10	8
Mother dead	0	2
Total	10	10
Schooling:		
Illiterate	4	1
1st grade	4	3
2nd grade	2	3
3rd grade	—	2
4th grade	—	1
Total	10	10
Had suffered violent punishment	8	7
Conduct accepted at home	2	3
Total	10	10
Close relatives with mental illness	7	4
Close relatives without mental illness	3	6
Total	10	10
Economic difficulties at home	8	7
No economic difficulties at home	2	3
Total	10	10
Alcoholic father	5	5
Nonalcoholic father	5	5
Total	10	10
Alcoholic mother	3	4
Nonalcoholic mother	7	6
Total	10	10

Table 1 (Continued).

Characteristics	Number of Gamines	Number of Nongamines
Stepfather or step- mother at home	2	1
Single-parent home	4	8
Completely broken home	1	—
Home with both parents	3	1
Total	10	10

Discussion by Chester M. Pierce, M.D.

In the near future, psychiatry and many other disciplines will be obliged to consider the type of material presented here. Among the issues that impressed me were: (1) how antichild social pressures force youngsters to extreme stress, (2) how resilient, adaptive, and resourceful these youngsers are in the face of such stress, and (3) how necessary it will be to gather long-range, cross-cultural, longitudinal studies of street children from all over the globe.

Dr. Gutierrez has presented a methodology which can be scrutinized as we search for models to engage these broad issues. It would seem incontestable that some sort of "outreach" will be required and that investigators must win legitimacy in the eyes of their subjects, just as Dr. and Mrs. Gutierrez did. Similarly, data collected must be guided by participants and the researchers must consider unconscious psychological forces. The accomplishment of these conditions will present major research problems.

In the present study I am sure the author is aware of deficiencies in the research which reflect probably the difficulty of working in the field. For instance, the efforts at making a matched control are heroic but the text fails to indicate how congruent each subject was to his matched partner. Thus although we may know that 3 gamines and 4 nongamines were children of urban fathers, we are not certain that these same 7 children are those who completed a first-grade education.

Another problem in data interpretation doubtlessly reflects the brevity of time allowed for presentation. I think most readers would like to know just what sort of questionnaire instrument was used, how the sample was selected, what universe it represented, and how Freudian theory was utilized in data analysis. Most readers will also wish the author had had time to present more clinical material about the individual lives of the gamines and will wish to know how he formulates their psychodynamics.

There will be an ever-increasing number of social scientists who will applaud efforts by analysts to move beyond the confines of the consultation room and into the area of action research and social advocacy. Hopefully, the applause will be even greater if it seems that the investigators are seen as creditable by their subjects and yet can maintain some sort of objective rigor and meticulous scholarhip on which they base their suggestions for social change. Regrettably, before such applause becomes commonplace we can anticipate many replications of the sort of personal suffering and anguish that plagued Dr. Gutierrez and his family.

From my own experience working with teen-age gangs in New York after World War II, I am able to look at specific individuals who now are adults. Probably the great bulk of them are functioning, contributing citizens. A good proportion have had higher education. Many have been very active in the social struggles of our time. However, in reading this paper I considered what will become of the Colombian gamine since it may be that comparatively he will have less education, more isolation from potentially helpful adults, even less benefits from an economy geared to exclude persons with his background, and probably equal if not greater political and social upheaval in his country. We might predict too that if social conditions intensify the hardships for the gamines, there will result increasing violence both specifically and nonspecifically directed, as they give bent to the frustrations and harshness of their lives. It seems amazing that even now under such powerful duress there is so little described violence and bitterness. The ridicule and arrogance now exhibited to adults may harden to more routine primitive, brutal expressions if the gamines' life burdens are not relieved.

Such relief depends on knowledge gained under the aegis of the intellectual humility and human-heartedness as reported in this paper. Novel methods, now either unknown or considered exotic in the therapeutic armamentarium of psychiatrists, must be wed with the fraction of truth known by clinicians from their understanding of the unconscious and their grasp of the dynamics of human behavior. Then, at best, we will be able to help gamines and street children all over this earth. At the least we'll know (just as in the paper under consideration) that some gamines have lived a bit better, with fuller, more dignified experiences for having had the privilege of knowing a therapist. And I suspect that therapists will have lived a bit better, with fuller, more dignified experiences from having had the privilege of knowing the children of the streets.

Cognitive Adaptation: A Mental Retardation Research Project

YASUHIKO TAKETOMO, M.D.

The Cognitive Development Service, Bronx State Hospital, is an innovative service for the treatment of, and research into, ways of altering the status of cognitively handicapped long-time residents of the state hospital system. Our immediate target group is those adult retarded who have a history of psychoses or psychotic episodes. [1]

As a research problem, in the usual sense of objective-reductive research, the question of mental retardation is as challenging as any other major question in medicine. Laboratories such as the one at the Kennedy Center for Research in Human Development and Mental Retardation are actively engaged in fundamental research, employing highly specialized techniques.

In the research orientation of our service, we are also engaged, within the reductive-objective frame of reference, in an interdisciplinary diagnostic approach, partly in affiliation with the Kennedy Center, and partly in conjunction with other research projects in preparation or under way.

Our research in this condition of cognitive dysfunction, however, has not kept us from realizing that, basically, we must know our patients as individuals rather than simply in reductionistic terms. Siirala[2] wrote:

Human life, community life, is so structured that a defect does not as such, and without much ado, imply misfortune or impoverishment for the individual or the community. Nor does it from the point of view of the defective person's self-recognition, his experience of himself, and his suffering of himself. The individual's happiness is in the continuous unfolding of his experience, and also in the fruitfulness of his suffering. The criterion of his happiness is his power and permission to grow into his own self, and all that it involves. This in turn, depends on other circumstances: the reality or mere ostensibility of his reception: the degree to which he is allowed, together with his defects and inherited birth constellations, to become integrated into his community, and the degree to which the community is permitted to become integrated into what he, the individual, represents.

Siirala does not advocate the professional's suppression of his recognition of the limited adaptational capacity of the defective person; rather he points to the essential need for the professional to dissociate himself from any attitude of hopelessness:

From moment to moment, and from place to place, the direction of the process will be determined—even "decided"—by the extent to which the people whom the challenge is reaching can identify their own despair and discriminatory attitude, by how far they dare to struggle with these. Such identification again is only possible if there is hope; and hope cannot be patented, only cherished.

Identification of the defects cannot be achieved solely by labeling—e.g., in terms of IQ, or phenylketonuria. We also need to learn how to recognize and to draw on the adaptational features of the experiential (introspective) structures of the "defective" person; i.e., the introspective structure of the person's self-experience as available through communication and interaction. Our concern in dealing with a retarded person whose predominant problem is cognitive arrest or handicap entails bringing the self as a cognitive system to the foreground, as a target area of psychodynamic inquiry.

Although the cognitive aspect of total personality has tended to be neglected in psychodynamic development, Arieti's contributions[3-9] are a salient exception to this. Arieti's psychodynamic model, "intrapsychic self,"[7-9] is presented in a highly condensed form in Table 1.

The model is *genetic* in three senses:

1. It is *ontogenetic* (or *epigenetic*) as shown in the stages that I have shown as I through V.

2. It is *phylogenetic*, in the sense that the model was formed partly in reference to the evolutional sequence of cognitive development.

3. It provides the context for *microgenetic* considerations. Microgeny

has to do with the immediate unfolding of a phenomenon—that is, the sequence of those steps that are inherent in the psychological process.

Further, the model is *systematic* in the sense that it traces major systems of the introspective experiences (cognition, emotion, self, etc.) in their respective modes of epigenesis and correlates them with corresponding levels of epigenesis. The systems tend to differentiate themselves from the global conglomerate as one traces each of them to more developed levels.

The stages of development of what I call "self-system" (the first column next to "Stage" in Table 1) are defined by the mode of cognitive operations, as it determines the experience of self. Thus "primordial self," "self-image," "self-identity," and "self and guilt," in Arieti's context, are all experiences of the self in the cognitive modes of the respective stages.

Although independently developed, Arieti's model has striking similarity to what Rado[10-13] attempted to formulate with his psychodynamic model. The latter has to do with the hierarchy of the integrative system and the action self which "at psychodynamic levels of the hierarchy of integration comes to represent the total organism in action. As the highest controlling unit of the integrative apparatus, the action-self must be located axially to the four units i.e., the levels of integration previously described, occupying the central position in each of them."

Rado's four units or levels include hedonic self-regulation, preverbal brute emotion, emotional thought, and unemotional thought. These, in turn, closely parallel stages I to V, respectively, in Arieti's model. It was Arieti's vigorous study of the cognitive aspect that led to his differentiation of III and IV, which is not to be found in Rado.

In the self-system, also, both Arieti and Rado start with what they call "primordial self," although there is some uncertainty whether Rado extended his primordial self to the hedonic control level—as in Fig. 2 of his paper[12]—or whether, like Arieti, he regarded its emergence as taking place at the level of brute emotion, as one would surmise from the text of his papers. While Arieti discusses the "discrepancy between the way one feels he is and the way one feels he should be," Rado introduces the concepts of "tested self" and "desired self." Arieti's differentiation of the stages of the self-system and of the corresponding cognitive modes considerably clarifies what Rado meant when he stated "the action-self must be located axially to the four units."

Because they formulated these models while working primarily with neurotics, psychotics, and psychopaths, neither of these workers seems to have applied his model to the condition of arrest of cognitive development: mental retardation.

Since our retarded patients are most seriously handicapped in verbal communication, various modes of nonverbal remedial methods are being researched at our service. These include: music therapy, dance therapy, occupational therapy, art therapy, recreational therapy, behavior modification therapy, and nursing programs. Some observations made during these remedial procedures are germane to the subject under consideration.

*Example:** Josephine, 43 yr. old, and with the mental age of 1:06–2:00, came to us from another unit, where she had been tied to a wheel chair because of her history of seizures, her occasional hyperactivity, and the consequent fear that she might fall on her face. Her feet did not touch the ground during all that time. When dance therapy was started, she had to be assisted to the dining room; she had no sense of weight or center of gravity. Soon, however, Josephine was able to walk in a side-to-side manner. Her eye contact initially was blank, with a fixed stare. The therapist worked for 4 mo. with her, doing such things as bilateral, controlled, alternating creeping. Although Josephine had little strength at the beginning, she now became able to pick up a ball and throw it a long distance and to join group sessions. She often talks to staff and others saying, "Hello, Honey," or speaks in an unintelligible language, apparently a derivative of Italian.

In effect, Josephine's mode of adaptation to her previous environment had been such as to induce occasional hyperactivity; this was interfered with by the external force of fixing her in a wheel chair, without her feet touching the step. What we inferred from observations made during the initial phase of her presence in our service was severe disturbance in the experience of motor identity and in awareness of the totality of self—the two components of the primordial self.

Her transfer to the service induced many changes in her adaptation (in the sense of bilateral encounter, not unilateral adjustment) vis-a-vis the environment (*Umwelt*). One of the significant experiences in this regard was her meetings with the dance therapist who, throughout the many months of dyadic interaction, induced the patient to experience an array of her own elementary movement perceptions in interacting with the environment. Viewed within the psychodynamic context, dance therapy had as its direct target repair and development of the primordial self.

It was with this repair successfully in progress (Josephine started voluntary ambulation) that her environment (*Umwelt*) became definitely widened and differentiated (ambulation and throwing balls); moreover, the burgeoning of her social activity (coming to join the group session) suggested the active formation of images on her part. At this point, one might assume that she is in stage III (self-image); yet her vocal activity, as well as what may be sufficiently complex linguistic activity, suggests that she is now thinking in terms of "I" and "you"— that is, that she is at stage IV of the self-system.

What we are describing may be simply symptomatic rather than curative changes, but we are not as yet in a position to attribute these changes

These data are based on the direct observations of Mrs. Susan Brainard, dance therapist of our service.

solely to the dance therapy, since Josephine was also receiving sensory training by an occupational therapist and interacting with other members of her environment during the same period. Even at this preliminary stage of the program, however, it is to be noted that our nonverbal approaches are directed toward those aspects of experience that are relevant to the more primordial levels of the "self-system"—e.g., integration of movement patterns; and references to the private space (bodily axes) of movements and posture, to the gravitational field, and to public space (territoriality and other aspects of *Umwelt*).

There has recently developed an interest among occupational, educational, and physiotherapists in linking primitive motor responses with higher cognitive functions (Kessler,[14] pp. 138–146). On the remedial side, perceptual-motor training has been advocated, and on the theoretical side, the concepts of body image and "self-system" are seen as pivotal. Concerning the more conceptualized experience of the "self-system," a concise review of contemporary research pertaining to the retarded person's experience of self can be found in Bialar.[15] This review covers the conception of self, conception of others (perception of other retardates, of nonretarded peers, and of "significant others"), and the projected self-percept. These "phenomenological variables" are relevant social-psychological factors in our consideration of the "self-system" at the verbal levels of IV or V. What led us to change the name of our service from Mental Retardation Service to Cognitive Handicap Service and finally to Cognitive Development Service was our finding strong refutations of the "identity of mental retardation" among some of our verbal patients. Dealing with the retarded person without verbal communication necessarily gives rise to an examination of the nature of the more primordial layers of the "self-system."

It is expected that availability for the retarded of the higher levels of the "self-system" may be limited in ways that are individually determined and in which, with severely and profoundly retarded persons, we are able to see the dynamic interrelations between the more primordial levels more clearly than we can elsewhere. The case given above exemplifies the care that we have to take before arriving at the conclusion that an adult person has, ontogenetically speaking, *never* reached the verbal stage IV.

Our daily encounter with a patient brings us into direct contact with the adaptive levels of the ongoing portion of his life that characterize his self-system. Our conceptual approach, in employing Arieti's model, is not to regard a person's self-system as being fixated (or arrested) rigidly at one of the levels, but rather to conceive it as shifting from level to level, in a way that is analogous to the levels of temporality of internal experience, as discussed elsewhere (Taketomo,[16] especially Fig. 1, p. 121).

Table 1. A Paradigm of Arieti's Psychodynamic Model, "Intrapsychic Self"

Stage	Self-System	Cognition	Emotion
I		*Sensation perception (immediate)*	*Feeling* (awareness, subjectivity) with pleasant/unpleasant tonality
II	*Primordial self*: Motor identity and awareness of totality of body	*Sensation perception (distant)*: Without a definite distinction of part/whole	*Protoemotion* (1st-order emotion): Tension, fear, rage; appetite, satisfaction
		Exocept (= engram): Representation of perception subsequently embodied in movement	
III	*Self-image*: A group of faceless images determined by the wishes	*Images*: Quasi reproduction of perception without requiring stimulus for evocation	*2nd-order emotion*: Anxiety; wish
		Paleosymbol: Image linked privately to an external counterpart	*Endocept*: Nonrepresentational, preverbal, vague emotion that may be retained in memory and later translated into "surprise," "doubt," "solemnity," etc., postulated as source of empathy and intuition

Cognitive processes are characterized by: (1) lack of causality; (2) lack of ego boundary, (3) possibility of transfer of past and future

Preparatory stages of symbolic externalization: (1) Finger pointing, (2) gesture, (3) vocalization: (a) word of action, (b) imperative verb, (c) primitive word, (d) denotation, (e) opposite use of words

Table 1 (Continued)

Stage	Self-System	Cognition	Emotion
IV	*Self-identity:* Not only a group of images, but also a name, or "I"; this self may undergo metamorphosis in accordance with wish and fear	*Paleologic organization:* Initial stage of connotation which is characterized by identification by predicate (Von Domarus); cognitive process is characterized by primary process features (Freud), anthropomorphic causality, and endocentrism (Piaget) Objects may be internalized, partially abstracted—paleologic metamorphosis—and projected The past and nonimmediate future emerge as full temporal dimension Verbal sequencing of events is possible	*3rd-order emotion:* Depression, hate; joy, love
V	*Self:* No longer a physical entity or a name but a repository of concepts which refer to his own person *Guilt:* Experience of discrepancy between the way one feels he is and the way one feels he should be	*Aristoteliam conceptual organization:* Development of this organization follows six stages: from motor-affective syncretic concept, to clear abstract relational concept without accessory connotation The higher-level cognitive process is characterized by induction, deduction, and deterministic causality Clear mental structure emerges concerning future time, conception of future, and of the possible	

Derived from Arieti.[7]

Psychodynamic inquiry into cognitive adaptation in neuroses and psychoses has dealt primarily with the elucidation of the dynamic relations between levels IV and V. Although the limited verbal communication in work with retarded persons obliges us to be reserved about the inferences we make, an opportunity is here provided of a new approach to a consideration of primordial stages, such as II and III, which are passed through all too hurriedly during normal development.[7]

References

1. Taketomo, T.: The Mentally Retarded Adult with Psychotic Phases. Presented at the V World Congress of Psychiatry, Mexico City, Mexico, Nov. 28–Dec. 4, 1971.
2. Siirala, M.: Medicine in Metamorphosis: Speech, Presence and Integration. London, Tavistock Publications, 1969.
3. Arieti, S.: Schizophrenia: The manifest symptomatology, the psychodynamics and normal mechanism. In: Arieti, S. (Ed.): American Handbook of Psychiatry, Vol. L. New York, Basic Books, 1959, pp. 455–484.
4. Arieti, S.: The microgeny of thought and perception. Arch. Gen. Psychiat. 6:494, 1962.
5. Arieti, S.: Contributions to cognition from psychoanalytic theory. In: Masserman, J. (Ed.): Communication and Community, Vol. VIII of Science and Psychoanalysis. New York, Grune & Stratton, 1965, pp. 16–37.
6. Arieti, S.: Conceptual and cognitive psychiatry. Amer. J. Psychiat. 122:361–366, 1965.
7. Arieti, S.: The Intrapsychic Self: Feeling, Cognition and Creativity in Health and Mental Illness. New York, Basic Books, 1967.
8. Arieti, S.: The role of cognition in the development of inner reality. In: Hellmuth, J. (Ed.): Cognitive Studies, Vol. I. New York, Brunner/Mazel, 1970.
9. Arieti, S.: The structural and psychodynamic role of cognition. In: Arieti, S. (Ed.): The World Biennial of Psychiatry and Psychotherapy, Vol. I. New York, Basic Books, 1971, pp. 3–33.
10. Rado, S.: Emergency behavior: With an introduction to the dynamics of conscience. In: Hoch, P. H., and Zubin, J. (Eds.): Anxiety (the proceedings of the 39th Annual Meeting of the American Psychopathological Association, New York City, June, 1949). New York, Grune & Stratton, 1950.
11. Rado, S.: Hedonic control, action-self, and the depressive spell. In: Hoch, P. H., and Zubin, J. (Eds.): Depression (the proceedings of the 42nd Annual Meeting of the American Psychopathological Association, New York City, 1953). New York, Grune & Stratton, 1954.
12. Rado, S.: From the metapsychological ego to the bio-cultural action self. J. Psychol. 46:279–285, 1958.
13. Rado, S.: Adaptational psychodynamics: Motivation and control. In: Jameson, J., and Klein, H. (Eds.): New York, Science House, 1969.
14. Kessler, J. W.: Contributions of the mentally retarded toward a theory of cognitive development. In: Hellmuth, J. (Ed.): Cogn tive Studies, Vol. I. New York, Brunner/Mazel, 1970, pp. 111–209.

15. Bialar, I.: Emotional disturbance and mental retardation: Etiologic and con-conceptual relationships. In: Menolascino, F. J. (Ed.): Psychiatric Approaches to Mental Retardation. New York, Basic Books, New York, 1970, pp. 68–90.
16. Taketomo, Y.: Levels of temporality in psychopathology. In: Arieti, S. (Ed.): The World Biennial of Psychiatry and Psychotherapy, Vol. I. New York, Basic Books, 1970, pp. 112–150.

Discussion by Silvano Arieti, M.D.

Dr. Taketomo's schema of personality that he derived from my book *The Intrapsychic Self* is not only accurate and complete in its brevity, but also an example of clarity.

Unfortunately, until very recently psychiatry and psychoanalysis have ignored cognition, but the psychiatrist who is willing to explore the field will not find complexities or obscurities such as are tied in with concepts such as cathexis, counter-cathexis, neutralization, bound energy, and energetics. The subject matter will appear easy to assimilate once reluctance is overcome.

I appreciated Dr. Taketomo's attempt to compare my theoretical framework to that of Sandor Rado. Taketomo thus joins the number of people who have studied cognition not merely as a way to deal with the external world, but also as a builder of the inner life, or as the major component of the self-image and of the self. Although it would be incorrect to minimize the contributions of Piâget and of other academic psychologists, we must recognize that they have dealt predominantly with the cognition of the secondary process, not of the primary, not with what is psychodynamically significant for psychic reality and therefore of major concern to a psychiatrist and psychoanalyst. The psychologist Heinz Werner, with his comparative developmental approach, is an important exception.

Taketomo follows Siirala in not considering the cognitive defect purely in a negative way, but in interpreting it psychodynamically and in visualizing the possibility of a rewarding human life in spite of it. Although Taketomo's application of psychodynamic cognition to the field of mental retardation is still at its beginning, it appears to be a prelude to important and extensive work.

part 3

PSYCHODYNAMIC RESEARCH

A Research Approach to the Imperative
Idea and Dream*

ARTHUR W. EPSTEIN, M.D.

An imperative idea[1] or dream may be defined as one which appears in forced and repetitive fashion and is of unvarying content. How does one define an idea? A definition offered by Webster is: "A representation or construct of memory and association as distinguished from direct impression of sense." How a dream? Not entirely differently—dreams are the ideas occurring during sleep, and their unique characteristics are shaped by this fact. Ideas often contain a feeling tone: pleasure or pain. Further, since ideas are mental internalizations of experiences with objects or events, an approach or avoidance posture may also be part of their structure. An idea endowed with pleasurable feeling tone has an approach valence, but if endowed with painful feeling tone, an avoidance valence. Of course, many ideas may be devoid of or have lost such feeling tone or valence.

An idea which is forced and repetitive is by definition not subject to usual control mechanisms. A state of dyscontrol exists[2] permitting the idea to make its appearance. Here a distinction between the waking and sleeping idea must be made. By their nature, dreams appear involuntarily

*This study was supported in part by U.S. Public Health Service Grant 5 R01-MH13918.

and are not subject at least to volitional control. However, when a dream appears overly repetitively, it, too, might be considered a product of discontrol. In contrast, in the waking state, ideas are more subject to voluntary control and selection.

If waking or sleeping ideas exist in a state of discontrol, one may postulate an impairment in the mechanisms of mind. Next, one may be permitted the speculation that there is an impairment in the substratum of mind; in short, a pathophysiology of the brain exists. That this assumption is not too speculative and is amply supported by clinical evidence is shown, for example, by the appearance of waking repetitive forced ideas[3, 4] and of dreams[5-8] as seizure components in temporal lobe epilepsy. The accumulation of such clinical data is in keeping with the statement made by Hughlings Jackson in 1875[9] concerning the appearance of mental automatisms in epileptic states: "The mental automatism results, I consider, from overaction of lower nervous centers, because the highest or controlling centers have been thus put out of use." In essence, Jackson states, "There is (1) loss of control permitting (2) increased automatic action." It would seem that the epileptic model, in both its clinical and electroencephalographic aspects, may serve as a research approach to the phenomenon of the imperative idea and dream. As encountered clinically, the imperative dream is known as the recurrent dream and the imperative idea as, among others, the obsessional, fetishistic, and phobic idea.

Imperative dreams

In clinical epileptics. Although Jackson described complex mental states occurring during daytime uncinate (temporal lobe) seizures and considered them "dreamy states," he made little mention of a possible relationship between such states and nocturnal dreams nor did he study nocturnal dreams. It remained for Penfield and co-workers[5, 10] to demonstrate the relationship between nocturnal dreams and seizures both through clinical case taking and electrical stimulation of the exposed temporal cortex. Penfield demonstrated in certain patients identical content in both nocturnal dreams and daytime temporal lobe seizures; he postulated that seizure content and dream "depend on the same neuronal mechanism in the temporal cortex."[10]

More recent work has corroborated the studies of Jackson and Penfield and has particularly established a relationship between recurrent dreams and temporal lobe seizures.[6-8] This relationship may assume varied forms.[6] (1) A dream appearing recurrently for some time may eventually become part of a daytime seizure. (2) A recurrent dream, identical in content to a daytime seizure, may appear concurrently with the seizure either independently or as a seizure component. (3) Recurrent dreams may appear simultaneously with seizures, but not necessarily becoming actual seizure components or even related in content to them. (4) Recurrent dreams may occur at some point in the lives of individuals with temporal lobe seizures, but apparently unrelated to the seizures either in time or in manifest content.

It may be of value to provide illustrations of the first three relationships.[6] In the first, a man has a recurrent stereotyped dream of falling, painful in feeling tone, occurring over a time span of 16 yr. For the next 5 yr, the dream begins to appear intrusively during the day. Finally, on one occasion, the daytime appearance of the dream is followed immediately by loss of consciousness and a generalized convulsion. Clearly, the dream is part of an epileptic process. In similar cases[10, 11] the content of frightening recurrent dreams which also made their appearance during the day is followed by evident epileptic manifestations, reflecting an actual frightening life event—that is to say, the ideation reappearing as part of the epileptic process represents the memory of a frightening event.

As an illustration of the second relationship,[6] a woman has seizures whose content contains the painful image of herself being drowned or trapped by fire; frequent dreams, appearing concurrently, have an identical content. It is noted that, in childhood, an actual attempt was made on this woman's life by drowning. To illustrate situation 3,[6] a woman reported the simultaneous appearance of temporal lobe seizures and recurrent frightening dreams. The seizures themselves did not contain ideational content, consisting only of visceral and *déjà vu* sensations. The dreams were of varied content but were uniformly painful in feeling tone. In all four relationships, the dreams have a fearful catastrophic quality. The ideation of the dream may have "typical" themes.

Clinical observations indicate that dream ideation in temporal lobe epileptics with recurrent dreams may be influenced in additional ways by the discharging focus. Disturbances in body image or position (falling or other movement), for example, may occur as part of the seizure and also in recurrent dreams.[8] Such a patient had a painful recurrent dream in which her mother and father were moving quickly toward her on different trains; this dream was linked with seizure phenomena involving body movement. Thus a sensation of body movement, presumed to reflect brain discharge, perhaps in temporal areas subserving vestibular input, may shape the nature of dream ideation.

In view of the relationship, observed clinically, between imperative dreams and seizures in certain epileptics, the question arises whether this relationship can be further demonstrated in an experimental situation. The avenue for such a demonstration is provided by the discovery of REM sleep and of the relationship of REM sleep to dreaming by Kleitman and Aserinsky.[12] Accordingly, all-night sleep studies with continuous electro-encephalographic recordings have been made on temporal lobe epileptics with recurrent stereotyped dreams. Among the many possible questions open to study in this situation are: whether dream ideation is consistently stereotyped; whether electroencephalographic abnormalities occur during the night's sleep, and, if so, whether such abnormalities are more pronounced during REM sleep; whether there is any correlation between an electroencephalographic abnormality during REM sleep, if it should occur, and the nature of dream ideation. In order to study these questions, criteria for patient selection should include not only an epileptic individual with recurrent dreams, but also one with a clear-cut electroencephalographic abnormality (usually prominent temporal spiking or slowing) to serve as a marker throughout the night's sleep.

A woman with painful recurrent dreams, often of a threatening nature (being attacked) and containing an epigastric sensation similar to that noted during daytime seizures, was studied for 2 nights in the sleep laboratory.[7] In all but one REM period, rhythmic continuous spiking was recorded from the right temporal area. Electroencephalographic abnormalities occurred during other sleep phases, but epileptiform spiking was confined to REM sleep. Whenever the patient was awakened from a REM period during which this right temporal spiking occurred (there were five such instances), an unpleasant dream along with an epigastric sensation was reported. An excerpt of such a dream is as follows: "I was talking to my cousin's wife, who is going to have a baby in four months. I saw my aunt coming. I got a nervous feeling in my stomach because she always wants to talk about babies." In this patient, dream ideation varied; the recurrent features were the epigastric sensation and the dysphoric quality of the dreams.

Among additional temporal lobe epileptics studied by means of all-night sleep recordings[13] are 2 who, by history, have recurrent dreams of dying and of being drowned, respectively. In these 2 patients, whose detailed data will be presented elsewhere, sustained and often rhythmic epileptiform abnormalities occur characteristically during REM sleep (Figs. 1 and 2). However, studies to date indicate that such an abnormality is not always correlated with the appearance of a recurrent dream since occasionally there may be either no dream recall or not the characteristic recurrent dream during the appearance of this abnormality in REM sleep.

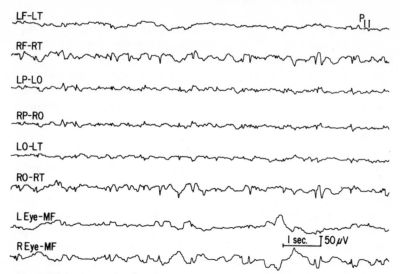

Fig. 1. Right temporal spike and slow activity, during REM sleep of a patient described in text. REM's are clearly shown in outer canthi leads. F = frontal, T = temporal, P = parietal, O = occipital. L and R indicate left and right sides, respectively. L eye is the left outer canthus with the midforehead (MF) as reference; R eye is the right outer canthus.

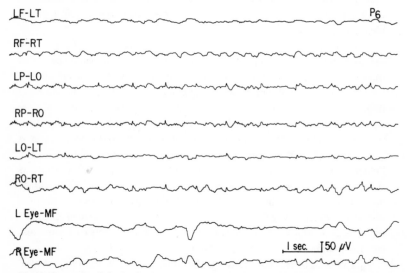

Fig. 2. Example of rhythmic right temporal slowing, best demonstrated in RF-RT line, during REM sleep of the same patient. REM's are clearly shown in outer canthi leads.

Therefore, although it is intriguing that sustained epileptiform abnormalities may occur during REM periods of epileptic patients with imperative dreams, a word of caution must be introduced for fear of making too sweeping a generalization in this regard. Indeed, one would be naïve always to anticipate a precise correlation between such an epileptiform abnormality and the imperative dream itself. However, when such an abnormality of sustained epileptiform type appears, it is hypothesized that dream content may then be affected.

How is dream ideation influenced in such epileptics? First, certain elements clearly related to the discharging neural focus may appear in the dream, for example, epigastric sensation and alteration in body image or position. Second, the stereotypy of image itself, for example, repeated dreams of dying, may be a reflection of discharge of a specific neural substratum during the epileptic process. There are undoubtedly other ways of influence as yet unknown. The role of a traumatic memory trace in influencing the imperative nature of the dream in certain epileptics has not been further enlarged to date by the all-night sleep studies. During the all-night sleep of some epileptics, REM awakenings yield "typical themes," for example, the self being endangered or dying. Whether or not such "typical themes" are related to a specific ontogenetic memory in the individual studied is not clear. It may also be mentioned that, in one individual, the content of a recurrent dream also appeared frequently as a forced idea during the day.[13]

In nonepileptics. A relationship between imperative dreams and temporal lobe epilepsy in certain individuals seems well established. The question next arises: what may be said of individuals with recurrent dreams who are not clinically epileptic? Immediately one is struck with inherent difficulties in unraveling this problem, for, as previous longitudinal case studies demonstrate, recurrent dreams may be the prelude to a frank epileptic disorder. How, then, can one tell whether the recurrent dream is or is not part of an epileptic process unless one knows the individual's entire life-span? Common sense and clinical experience indicate, however, that there must be individuals with recurrent dreams who never demonstrate clinical epilepsy. But here one may be dealing with a *forme fruste* of a disorder. Indeed, Savage,[14] as early as 1912, regarded as "masked epilepsy" those cases in which "the patient complains of the recurrence of some distressful dream, always of the same kind."

Of interest in this connection is the study of "typical dreams." As the name indicates, typical dreams seem to be universally experienced and include such dreams as: the self or other object dying or endangered, falling through space, being chased or attacked, being drowned, being exposed to fire, something happening to the teeth, being able to fly, and seeing snakes.[15,16] Typical dreams tend to be recurrent, easily recalled, and "resist interpretation by the usual association techniques."[15] The origin of typical dreams is an enigma. Freud[17] felt they represented infantile experiences of virtually universal occurrence. On the other hand, it is possible that such dreams may represent innate patterns of species-specific import.

Individuals with frequent typical dreams but without clinical epilepsy, when encountered and when agreeable to study, have slept in the all-night laboratory.[18] Of 4 individuals studied whose typical dreams, by history, were painful and frequent, 3 had abnormal wave forms in their all-night electroencephalograms although no sustained epileptiform abnormalities occurred. Although a stereotyped typical dream was reported on awakening from REM sleep in at least 1 of the patients, no sustained epileptiform abnormalities occurred during that REM period.

The varied contexts in which a typical dream may appear are noteworthy. In an individual with a "loss-of-teeth" dream, this dream, as determined from reports furnished on regular visits, was accompanied simply by a sensation in the mouth without other imagery or occurred in association with eating or erotic or being-attacked imagery. This indicates that the ideation of such a typical dream contains no single meaning but condenses many. This observation suggests that "typical" imagery has the capacity to be the carrier of various motivational states (wishes or fears) and also may occur as an isolated fragment associated only with a body sensation. It would seem that in certain individuals, there is a predilection for typical dream imagery to appear and that this imagery is linked to many other mental products. Is this due, one wonders, to a unique neurophysiological state in which this imagery is held?

Another example of the imperative dream in nonepileptics is the traumatic dream. The traumatic dream makes its appearance following an event of intense affect, usually marked fear, and essentially reproduces the event. At times one may see an exact duplication; at times some elaboration of the precipitating event. It has been indicated previously that events producing marked fear may initiate imperative dreams in certain temporal lobe epileptics and may also be duplicated in the seizure content. In such instances, one may presume that when in a pathophysiological state, the brain is likely to process an intensely affective event by automatically reproducing the event without its inhibition. However, imperative dreams may presumably occur in any individual who has been subjected to a fearful life-threatening event. Therefore, the "epileptic" brain is not a prerequisite for the appearance of the recurrent traumatic dream, but one is reasonably led to wonder whether events of a highly intense nature may produce a metabolic change in any brain; i.e., the neural substratum which must contain the memory of the event is rendered overly excitable.

The traumatic dream is a prominent symptom of the so-called war neurosis. Here death has stalked the environment and fear may be at its greatest. Several authors have reported the vivid and disturbing recurrent dreams of warfare. Rivers,[19] for example, described the recurrent appearance of the mangled, mutilated body of a fellow soldier in a patient's dream, which reproduced the real event of coming upon this soldier in the field. These dreams were of such intensity, in their reproduction of this disturbing episode, that the patient "dreaded to go to sleep." Rivers mentions the efficacy of abreaction in diluting and perhaps ultimately dissolving the tendency of these fearful dreams to return.

Imperative waking ideas

The obsessional idea in clinical epileptics. Ideas or ideational fragments may appear as a component of daytime seizures of temporal lobe epileptics. Appearing involuntarily, these ideas flood the field of consciousness, cannot be dispelled, and often have a painful feeling tone although, at times, they may be affect free. The ideas tend to arise endogenously, concurrent with the abnormal brain discharge, and are not necessarily precipitated by environmental stimuli.

The appearance of forced ideation as a temporal lobe seizure component has been studied by Hill and Mitchell.[3] These workers suggest that the perceptual-ideational seizure component changes over time. Early in the natural history of the seizure, a full-blown complex perceptual-ideational component may appear: for example, a visual scene, which often is a reduplication of an actual event. The event is often of significant affect, usually painful in feeling tone and occurring prior to the onset of the seizure disorder. Years later, only an isolated ideational fragment might appear during the seizure, but this fragment remains linked to the actual life event and is therefore part of a memory. The linkage between the fragment and the life event might be merely associative through various modes and need not carry the full affect of the original event. In seizure patients, the thought fragment appears involuntarily and is in some way linked to the seizure discharge due either to overactivity of a neural substratum and/or to impairment of inhibition normally exercised upon that substratum. The fate of these intrusive ideational fragments of the daytime seizure during sleep, for example, whether they appear in dreams, is not known since this type of epileptic has not been studied in the sleep laboratory nor are there adequate clinical reports of dream material.

The obsessional idea in nonepileptics. In the obsessional neurosis proper, an idea or idea fragment, often painful in feeling tone, appears intrusively during the waking state. The individual wishes to avoid the foreign painful idea. On the other hand, it is known from clinical studies that the individual may be drawn to the idea. There is then a combination of approach-avoidance tendencies, if you will, contained within certain obsessional ideas, particularly those of any complexity. Thus the obsessional idea "I fear I will kill someone by touching him" contains the wish to touch or kill the object (approach tendency) while at the same time there is an avoidance tendency reflecting the fear aspect. This is similar to the concept of Freud[20] that obsessional ideas represent "compromise formations." Containing opposite tendencies, obsessional ideas may have great condensation of meaning. The stereotyped recurrent idea may dominate waking conciousness and may, over the course of time, become the seed of numerous related ideas.

Although the great majority of individuals with obsessional ideas do not have clinical epilepsy, some have abnormal electroencephalograms. This is still a controversial point since routine waking electroencephalographic studies of obsessionals vary according to the series. Nevertheless, for example, Pacella et al.[21] reported waking electroencephalographic abnormalities, primarily generalized, in 20 of 31 patients with obsessional disorder.

When abnormal waking electroencephalograms in obsessional neurotics without clinical epilepsy are present, what is the fate of the abnormality during all-night sleep? A total of 14 nights of sleep was studied in 3 such individuals.[22] The electroencephalographic abnormalities of all 3 persist in sleep, but become more localized appearing over the temporal areas; they appear almost entirely during stage I and REM sleep and in a sporadic fashion. No sustained epileptiform abnormalities are noted. What is the ideation of these patients, upon awakenings from REM periods? In the patients studied, none of the dream ideation reported upon REM awakenings is identical to waking obsessional thoughts, but the imagery may be related. When sporadic abnormalities were present during individual REM periods, such abnormalities cannot be correlated with specific dream content. The electroencephalographic abnormalities bear some similarities to those of the temporal lobe epileptic in that a focal abnormality becomes manifest during sleep as contrasted to a normal or generalized abnormal pattern while awake. This all-night sleep study perhaps links the forced ideation of obsessional neurosis to the similar ideation occurring in certain temporal lobe seizures. Temporal (limbic) pathophysiology may exist in both.

The lack of identity between waking obsessional ideation and dream ideation is of interest. The painful affect of the waking obsessional thought is not reflected in the dream, in the 3 patients studied. Sleep seems to dilute the intensity of affect contained in the obsessional idea while awake. The complexity of the obsessional idea and its role of fusing conflicting approach-avoidance tendencies rather than representing a pure approach or pure avoidance pattern may require the capabilities of the waking state.

The fetishistic idea in clinical epileptics. In fetishism, an object evokes a sexual response of intense degree; a strong approach reaction develops. The image or idea of the object soon develops the attributes of the object itself. The image of the object often appears intrusively, almost always with pleasurable feeling tone, but because of its unbidden appearance, occasionally with painful feeling tone. The power of the fetish object or fetish image may in some instances persist for a lifetime.[23] Accumulated case studies indicate that the tenacious approach reaction (in effect, fusion) to the fetish begins early in life, perhaps in some "critical period" which helps bind this memory trace. As time progresses, the image of the fetish may be automatically employed to dispel both sexual and aggressive tensions.[24]

Fetishism in association with epilepsy, primarily temporal lobe epilepsy, has been reported.[25-27] There are various relationships between the fetish and seizures. The appearance of the fetish object, externally or in thought, may precipitate a seizure.[26] In the case of Mitchell, Falconer, and Hill,[26] the sense of pleasure evoked by the fetish was followed by a "blank period" and then, over the years, by the development of automatisms and other seizure phenomena. The subsequent accretion of epileptic symptomatology to the initial impairment of consciousness evoked by the fetish in this case suggests that the neural substratum related to the fetish complex has the capacity to recruit other neural areas.[28] It is of interest that fetishism has been reported abolished in 2 cases associated with temporal lobe epilepsy[26,27] by left anterior temporal lobectomy; in these instances gliosis was present in the anterior temporal region.

The fetishistic idea in nonepileptics. Although clinical epilepsy may be associated with fetishism, particularly temporal lobe epilepsy, the majority of fetishists do not present with a seizure picture. On the other hand, it is not uncommon for fetishists to have abnormal electroencephalograms, tending to implicate the temporal areas of the brain,[25, 23] and it has been suggested that temporal (limbic) pathophysiology may be the necessary "constitutional" factor underlying the genesis and persistence of the fetishistic symptom.[24, 28] Fetishism may be associated with other imperative ideas, both in waking and in dream states, not necessarily related to the fetish object.[24] The fetish object may appear repetitively in the dream imagery of clinical fetishists; its meaning in these instances is manifold. The fetish may appear as an isolated image in the dream, or in a clearly sexual context, or as part of some early memory, or as clearly symbolizing a body part.[23] When appearing in a dream, the image is frequently accompanied by a seminal emission. Thus, there appears to be an identity between the appearance of the fetish idea in waking or sleeping mentation; in both instances, the image is accompanied by sexual excitement. The condensation of meaning contained within the fetish image in the dream is paralleled in waking life. This is well expressed by Payne[29]: "Every component of the infantile sexual instinct has some connection with the fetish object." Study of all-night sleep in fetishists, whether clinically epileptic or not, has not as yet been done nor is it reported in the literature.

The phobic idea in clinical epileptics. There are no well-documented associations between phobic states and epileptic activity of the brain, although it is well known that the unpleasant feeling tone and avoidance patterns of fear itself are commonly encountered in temporal lobe epilepsy particularly in abnormal discharge of the anterior temporal region.

The phobic idea in nonepileptics. In phobic states, the phobic idea is almost always prompted by an external stimulus. One is therefore dealing primarily with an imperative response rather than an endogenously occurring imperative idea. Of interest, however, is the power of this response in that it may become generalized to many objects or situations related in some fashion to the one initially feared. The phobic idea is attended by painful emotion (fear) and therefore by an avoidance reaction. It is known, however, that occasionally an individual will be drawn to the phobic object or its internalization, the phobic idea, indicating some conversion of the avoidance to an approach reaction and possibly the introduction of a pleasurable emotion.

Of interest in phobic states is the mode of onset. Lief[30] has shown that the sensory context in which the initial fear attack occurs is of great importance in establishing the phobic symptom. The subsequent phobic response persists over time, although the initial sensory association may become fragmented or obscured. It is of interest that the persistent intrusive memories which are part of temporal lobe seizure content[3] may also represent a fearful external event; the seizure will then reduplicate time and time again the image of that event albeit a fragmentary image.

It is known that the dreams of phobics may have imagery similar, if not identical, to the waking phobic fear. Indeed, recurrent dreams in general have a phobic quality although they do not necessarily occur in individuals who have waking phobias. However, the fact that recurrent dreams similar or identical to the waking phobia may occur in patients with phobic states is of theoretical interest suggesting that a neural substratum is held in common and gains expression during both waking and sleeping states. Indeed, Silverman and Geer[31] report the elimination of a recurrent nightmare by desensitization of only a waking phobia but one with related imagery. Desensitization was achieved by having the individual visualize the frightening imagery while in a state of relaxation. Desensitization treatment may be viewed as one of controlled abreaction. It is known that abreaction is of importance in the treatment of phobias in general.

Discussion

What are some of the conclusions that can be drawn from the data?

Imperative ideas and dreams have certain common characteristics; they appear to be products of a disturbance in brain homeostasis. The epileptic state is the clearest example of such a disturbance and serves as a model for the study of these mental phenomena. The electroencephalogram is an important method of investigation in this model. At the current state of technological expertise, however, the electroencephalogram is able to detect only gross abnormalities; disturbance at subcortical levels may remain unrevealed. Further, one should not have overly naïve expectations of finding the neural substratum of an idea or dream. Indeed, what is meant by the neural substratum? One does not necessarily conceive of this as a well-defined anatomical entity but perhaps as a field effect or as-yet-unknown other process.

The data suggest that the degree of affect accompanying the initial perception of an event is of importance in establishing the future imperative idea or dream. The entire perceptual complex in which the affective event is experienced is significant since the associated perceptual material may later appear not only as part of the entire idea or dream itself, but as a fragment.

The time of life in which an event is experienced may be of importance, leading to consideration of the concept of a "critical period." The imperative idea of fetishism, for example, may take origin in a certain "critical period," although this is still speculative. The "critical period" may also apply to other clinical conditions in which the imperative idea or dream appears.

Perhaps not only is it necessary that an event of significant affect occur at a certain point in the life-span in order for an imperative idea or dream to be established, but there may be an innate factor favoring the establishment of ideas or dreams of certain content. Here one deals with species-specific or phylogenetic factors. For example, certain dream types may be more prone to become established as recurrent dreams due to species-specific factors. Similarly, certain situations leading to phobic ideas may be favored by a species-specific factor,[32] and certain attributes of the future fetish object may have species-specific significance.[23, 28]

Factors favoring establishment of the future imperative idea or dream not only may include the nature of an event, its time of appearance, and its possible species-specific import but also may be related to the physiological state of the brain at the time of a given event. In individuals who develop imperative ideas or dreams, there may at a given time be a certain metabolic state of the brain, which favors the engramming of the event in such a way that it is not subject to usual orderly processing. Also, of course, one must consider the possibility that any event of sufficiently intense affect may in itself influence brain metabolic processes in such a way that its processing is impaired.

Once established, the permanence and intrusive quality of the imperative idea or dream may well be related to the conditions of initial processing of this trace and may reflect, as is suggested, some neurophysiological irregularity.[33] The permanence and intrusiveness of these ideas, as reflecting a unique neural substratum, are similar to the concept of the self-continuing, closed, reverberating circuit proposed by Kubie.[34]

Once established, the imperative idea or dream tends to become dominant. Its dominance is already attested to by its intrusiveness (its abrupt appearance in a state of dyscontrol), but another characteristic of dominance is the tendency of the imperative idea or dream to become the nucleus of other ideas or images. The multiple condensation contained within a recurrent "typical" dream image (loss-of-teeth image) or fetish image is an example of a nucleus through which various motivational states or affects are expressed. The capacity to generalize, as is particularly true of obsessional and phobic ideas, is another attribute of such a nucleus. One may speculate that dominance is related to neurophysiological pecularities; the appropriate neural substratum has the capability of exciting or recruiting other neural substrata.

The dominance of the imperative idea or dream may be reduced by abreaction; that is to say, through expressing the duplication of its content and affect. This, of course, is a well-recognized psychological principle. It is suggested that the abreactive process in some way influences the neural substratum of the imperative idea or dream. Abreaction, of course, can be achieved in a normal state of consciousness or by means of hypnotic or drug-induced alterations in consciousness.

Certain imperative ideas may not be significantly modified by sleep. In the case of the fetishistic or phobic idea, for example, both may appear unchanged in waking and sleeping ideation (dreaming). However, in sleep, there may be further weakening of inhibition (impaired repression); for example, the phobic idea may be more vividly and terrifyingly expressed and there may be greater ease of seminal emission accompanying the appearance of the fetishistic idea. In a few instances, imperative dreams may appear, essentially unchanged, during the waking state—in which case they appear related to a frank epileptic process. However, another imperative idea, namely the obsessional idea, does not seem to be identically expressed in the sleeping state—at least not in the few cases studied. There may not be enough energy available at the level of dream ideation to duplicate the complicated obsessional idea of the waking state. The obsessional idea is not as concrete and cannot be as easily encompassed visually as the fetish or phobic image.

Imperative dreams are subject to influences which do not affect waking ideas. The idea in sleep may be more obviously molded by such factors as the physiological condition of the brain or other organs. Excitation of brain areas, for example, subserving visceral sensation or body image, may influence and become a recurrent feature of dream content. Sleeping mentation thus seems more subject to internal influences—which help to shape the imperative dream.

The element of inhibition or repression is of importance in any discussion of imperative ideas or dreams. As noted, there is weakening of repressive forces during the dream. The very nature of imperative ideas also indicates a weakening of repressive forces during the waking state. Paradoxically, the power of the imperative idea or dream is diluted in some instances, when remaining repression over the idea or dream is removed. This is illustrated by the reduction of the imperative ideas and dreams of the war neurosis when these are abreacted. This point was originally made by Breuer and Freud,[35] whose comments on the effect of their psychotherapeutic procedure may be recalled: "It brings to an end the operative force of the idea which was not abreacted in the first instance, by allowing its strangulated affect to find a way out through speech; and it subjects it to associative correction by introducing it into normal consciousness (under light hypnosis) or by removing it through the physician's suggestion, as is done in somnambulism accompanied by amnesia."

Finally, one should not conceive of imperative ideas or dreams as arising entirely from external events. Certainly the inner motivational system with its assigning of pain and pleasure to thought content may generate imperative ideas or dreams—although even here unique neurophysiological factors may be at work. However, a complete study of imperative ideas or dreams including their role in personality function lies beyond the scope of the present paper.

References

1. Tuke, D. H.: Imperative ideas. Brain 17:179–197, 1894.
2. Monroe, R. R.: Episodic Behavioral Disorders. Cambridge, Mass., Harvard University Press, 1970.
3. Hill, D., and Mitchell, W.: Epileptic anamnesis. Folia Psychiat. 56:718–725, 1953.
4. Brickner, R. M., and Stein, A.: Intellectual symptoms in temporal lobe lesions including "deja pensee." J. Mount Sinai Hosp. N. Y. 9:344–348, 1942.
5. Penfield, W., and Jasper, H.: Epilepsy and the Functional Anatomy of the Human Brain. Boston, Little, Brown and Co., 1954.
6. Epstein, A. W.: Recurrent dreams: Their relationship to temporal lobe seizures. Arch. Gen. Psychiat. 10:25–30, 1964.
7. Epstein, A. W., and Hill, W.: Ictal phenomena during REM sleep of a temporal lobe epileptic. Arch. Neurol. (Chicago) 15:367–375, 1966.
8. Epstein, A. W.: Body image alterations during seizures and dreams of epileptics. Arch. Neurol. (Chicago) 16:613–619, 1967.
9. Jackson, J. H.: In: Taylor, J. (Ed.): Selected Writings of John Hughlings Jackson. New York, Basic Books, 1958.
10. Penfield, W., and Rasmussen, T.: The Cerebral Cortex of Man. New York, Macmillan, 1950.
11. Kardiner, A.: The bio-analysis of the epileptic reaction. Psychoanal. Quart. 1:375–483, 1932.
12. Aserinsky, E., and Kleitman, N.: Two types of ocular motility occurring in sleep. J. Appl. Physiol. 8:1–10, 1955.
13. Epstein, A. W.: Unpublished data.
14. Savage, G. H.: Some dreams and their significance. J. Ment. Sci. 58:407–411, 1912.
15. Ward, C. H., Beck, A. T., and Rascoe, E.: Typical dreams: Incidence among psychiatric patients. Arch. Gen. Psychiat. (Chicago) 5:606–615, 1961.
16. Griffith, R. M., Miyagi, O., and Tago, A.: The university of typical dreams: Japanese vs. Americans. Amer. Anthropologist 60:1173–1179, 1958.
17. Freud, S.: The Interpretation of Dreams. New York, Basic Books, 1955.
18. Epstein, A. W.: Unpublished data.

19. Rivers, W. H. R.: Instinct and the Unconscious. Cambridge, England, Cambridge University Press, 1920.
20. Freud, S.: Notes upon a case of obsessional neurosis. In: Collected Papers, Vol. 3. London, Hogarth Press, 1950, pp. 293–383.
21. Pacella, B. L., Polatin, P., and Nagler, S. H.: Clinical and EEG studies in obsessive-compulsive states. Amer. J. Psychiat. 100:830–838, 1944.
22. Epstein, A. W., and Bailine, S. H.: Sleep and dream studies in obsessional neurosis with particular reference to epileptic states. Biol. Psychiat. 3:149–158, 1971.
23. Epstein, A. W.: Fetishism: A comprehensive view. In: Masserman, J. H. (Ed.): Dynamics of Deviant Sexuality, Vol. XV of Science and Psychoanalysis. New York, Grune & Stratton, 1969, pp. 81–87.
24. Epstein, A. W.: Fetishism: A study of its psychopathology with particular reference to a proposed disorder in brain mechanisms as an etiological factor. J. Nerv. Ment. Dis. 130:107–119, 1969.
25. Epstein, A. W.: Relationship of fetishism and transvestism to brain and particularly to temporal lobe dysfunction. J. Nerv. Ment. Dis. 133:247–253, 1961.
26. Mitchell, W., Falconer, M. A., and Hill, D.: Epilepsy with fetishism relieved by temporal lobectomy. Lancet 2:626–630, 1954
27. Hunter, R., Logue, V., and McMenemy, W. H.: Temporal lobe epilepsy supervening on longstanding transvestism and fetishism. Epilepsia 4:60–65, 1963.
28. Epstein, A. W.: The relationship of altered brain states to sexual psychopathology. In: Zubin, J., and Money, J. (Eds.): Critical Issues in Contemporary Sexual Behavior. Baltimore, Johns Hopkins Press. In press.
29. Payne, S. M.: Some observations on the ego development of the fetishist. Int. J. Psychoanal. 20:161–170, 1939.
30. Lief, H. I.: Sensory association in the selection of phobic objects. Psychiatry 18:331–338, 1955.
31. Silverman, I., and Geer, J. H.: The elimination of a recurrent nightmare by desensitization of a related phobia. Behav. Res. Ther. 6:109–111, 1968.
32. Marks, I. M.: Fears and Phobias. New York and London, Academic Press, 1969.
33. Epstein, A. W.: Contribution of epileptic phenomena to the study of memory mechanisms. Bull. Tulane Med. Fac. 25:305–309, 1966
34. Kubie, L. S.: Some implications for psychoanalysis of modern concepts of the organization of the brain. Psychoanal. Quart. 22:21–52, 1953.
35. Breuer, J., and Freud, S.: Studies on hysteria. In: Strachey, J. (Ed.): The Standard Edition of the Complete Psychological Works of Sigmund Freud, Vol. II. London, The Hogarth Press, 1955.

Suicide and Self-Destruction in Automobile Accidents: A Psychoanalytic Study*

NORMAN TABACHNICK, M.D.
CARL I. WOLD, PH.D.

The problem

Of what importance are psychological factors in the production of accidents, and specifically automobile accidents? The possibility that they are quite important has been considered in the literature of both psychology and research for many years. [1,2]

The impression has been supported by many anecdotal experiences of psychologists and psychoanalysts. [3] They have either heard patients report that their accidents have had psychological motivation or deduced such motivation from the nature of the events, the character of their patients, and their impression as to various drives within those patients.

Consider this case. A man of 48 had just been given an ultimatum by his mistress that he had to choose either his wife or her. He was in a depressed mood and was drinking at one of his usual haunts. While there, he discussed his problem with the bartender and a number of his cronies, giving numerous indications of the worthlessness of life and his feeling that suicide would be the only way to settle

*This work was supported by National Institute of Mental Health Grant MH-15510, administered through the University of Southern California.

his troubled feelings. Driving home, he had a one-car accident in which his car was completely demolished. He was not seriously injured and continued on to his home.

The next part of the story comes from his wife, who heard him enter the house. When he did not come into the bedroom after a few minutes, she went looking for him. She entered the living room just in time to see him shoot himself through the head and kill himself.

Impression: The "accident" was an attempt at suicide which failed and was then followed by a more successful attempt.

Within the last 10 yrs., there have been estimates that up to 80 percent of automobile accidents have a significant psychological factor.[4] Despite this, however, there has been a relative paucity of research which has elucidated exactly which psychological or psychopathological features may be important in understanding accidents. A number of factors which follow have contributed to this lack.

The Problem of Subject Selection

A major issue in current accident research is the selection of appropriate subjects. In a majority of studies done on psychology of accident victims, the target group studied has been those individuals who have actually been involved in accidents. The rationale is that if one can find certain characteristics in groups of subjects who have sustained accidents which are not present in nonaccident groups, such characteristics will help explicate the problem of accident.

In actual experience, such studies have not been greatly productive of valuable data. There are two factors that help explain this: (1) There is a relatively low accident rate for the population as a whole. (2) Most accidents are multifactorial in regard to cause. That is, in addition to whatever "psychological" factors may be operating, there are many additional ones. These have to do with the physical condition of the individual, factors affecting the performance of the vehicle, and a great number of factors outside of the vehicle such as the actions of other vehicles, climatic conditions, and highway conditions.

Because of these two circumstances (multi-factorial nature of accidents, and accident being a relatively rare occurrence), it is possible that many individuals who possess significantly high psychological accident-producing tendencies may *never* have an accident due to chance factors. Others whose psychological accident-producing tendencies are lower may (because of the many other factors which could produce an accident) have an accident.

Psychological Resistance

Another issue contributing to the determination of psychological factors highly correlated with accident can be called "psychological resistance." Many data in accident research are obtained from the victims or drivers of cars who have been involved in accidents. Yet there may be strong conscious or unconscious resistances operating which make these individuals give an essentially bland or false picture of what occurred during the period being researched.

With this as a background, let me now state the central purpose of our research. We wished to specifically study the question of whether there were suicide or suicide-like factors present to an increased degree in drivers who had involved their automobiles in accidents. In addition to this suicide hypothesis, we developed a number of other hypotheses referring to psychological self-destructive features in automobile drivers. Although the suicide hypothesis would, at best, have been important only in a certain subgroup of accident drivers, it was worth testing for the following reasons: (1) That such a group existed had been frequently postulated. (2) If, in fact, such a group did exist and could subsequently be identified, we would be availed of a body of knowledge (namely, that having to do with the treatment of suicide) which might be effective in preventing a certain proportion of automobile accidents. If any of the other self-destructive hypotheses proved to be supported, we would have valuable theoretical knowledge concerning the relationship of psychological factors in automobile accidents to the entire problem.

Method

The method we used had the following objectives:

We wished to study a series of psychodynamic psychoanalytic hypotheses in large enough comparison groups of individuals so that the results would have some statistical support.

We wanted to use psychoanalysts as the clinical investigators who obtained the data from the subjects. Our rationale was twofold: (1) the clinical skills of the psychoanalysts would enable them to dissipate some of the resistances which we anticipated would be forthcoming from the subjects. (2) The theoretical background and clinical experience of the psychoanalysts would enable them to make more accurate judgments on the pertinent research questions than would be possible for clinical investigators lacking specific psychoanalytic background and experience.

Our method proceeded by the following steps: First, we developed a series of hypotheses concerning suicide and self-destruction in serious automobile accidents. We then developed a data sheet which consisted of the following sections:

1. A series of 205 questions, each of which was related to one or more of the hypotheses.

2. A psychodynamic summary of pertinent events in the patient's life and particularly those parts of his life which surrounded his entry into the general hospital.

3. A discussion of the particular defenses and resistances which each subject utilized during his series of interviews.

In regard to the 205 items which constituted the first part of the data sheet, reliability of a high order was established by submitting taped interviews to raters and asking them to score the interviews for the 205 items. When items were found to have low reliability, they were revised until high reliability was achieved through further ratings. (These analyses were based on percentage of agreement among the raters on each item. Only items with at least 80 percent agreement were retained.)

In preparation for the research, we conducted a series of seminars which dealt with the theoretical background and the particular problems of interviewing subjects in a general hospital. The interviewers were all members of an advanced research seminar at the Southern California Psychoanalytic Institute. About half were psychoanalytic graduates; the others were people who all had had at least 3 yr. of psychoanalytic training.

The subjects were divided into three groups (all patients at a large general hospital in our area).

The serious accident group. These subjects were the drivers of cars that had been involved in one-car accidents. "Serious" was defined as requiring hospital stay and treatment of 2 or more days. We restricted the subjects to one-car accidents (which means that the driver's car hit an immobile object or overturned) because it was felt that it was in precisely such accidents that a maximalization of any suicidal or self-destructive psychological features would be found.

The suicide group. This group consisted of individuals who were in the hospital for treatment of severe suicide attempts ("severe" was defined as any patient who was hospitalized on the intensive care unit at any time, who was in coma at any time, or who was admitted to the ward, having been unconscious at least one-half hour any time prior to or during hospitalization).

The postappendectomy group. This group was chosen to represent individuals having an acute hospital experience for whom there is little in the psychological literature to suggest suicidal or self-destructive trends.

All subjects were males. From one standpoint, this was practically desirable since the majority of drivers involved in one-car accidents are men. There was an additional advantage in that we did not wish to add the additional variables which would be occasioned by having a bisexual sampling.

All subjects were between the ages of 18 and 48. A statistical evaluation showed that there were nonsignificant differences in regard to social class or age within the three groups.

Subjects were assigned to interviewers with the intent of minimizing the chances of any one interviewer getting a predominant number of subjects in any one category (accident, suicide, or appendectomy). Each interviewer was free to spend as much time as he wished, with a maximum of 10 hr., with each subject. The average amount of time spent was 3 hr. The analyst was allowed to conduct the interview in any way which was congenial to him, being asked only to report as much data as he could at the end of his series of interviews with each subject. The totality of each interview was tape recorded.

Hypotheses

At this point, let me list the specific hypotheses of our study. Drivers who sustain serious injury in automobile collisions:

1. Have utilized these collisions as deliberate suicide attempts to a greater degree than subjects in the appendectomy group.

2. Have made suicide attempts and communications of suicidal preoccupation to a greater degree than subjects in the appendectomy group.

3. Manifest depressive symptoms to a greater degree than subjects in the appendectomy group.

4. Manifest a counterdepressive attitude to a greater degree than subjects in the appendectomy group.

5. Indulge in excessive drinking and/or drug ingestion to a greater degree than subjects in the appendectomy group.

6. Tend to self-injuriously not seek and/or not follow medical advice to a greater degree than subjects in the appendectomy group.

7. Engage in behavior which risks injury or death to themselves to a greater degree than do subjects in the appendectomy group.

8. Have, in the period of 6 mo. prior to the accident, had unusual difficulty in dealing with a new responsibility to a greater degree than subjects in the appendectomy group.

9. Have a greater tendency than those in the appendectomy group to utilize impulsive actions which have a destructive implication.

10. Show a lack of integration between depressive, passive, inactive styles of life, on the one hand, and counter depressive, active, energetic styles of life, on the other hand, to a greater degree than subjects in the appendectomy group.

11. Will, just prior to their accidents, have suffered a loss of self-esteem to a greater degree than subjects in the appendectomy group.

12. In terms of a number of characteristics, those specified in hypotheses 2–11, drivers involved in serious accidents will be closer to a suicidal group than to those in the appendectomy group.

These hypotheses were developed from previous studies of the literature [5–7] as well as a number of previous accident studies which we ourselves had done. [8–10] The design of the study was to attempt to discover whether these hypotheses, all linked to self-destructiveness, would be manifested in a group of accident victims in a destribution that would be similar to that found in a group of suicide attempters and dissimilar to the distribution in a group of "normal" control subjects. If the accident victims were closer to the suicide attempters in terms of these hypotheses, then we would conclude that the hypothesis was supported, and that these supposed correlates of self-destruction and suicide were present in our group of accident subjects. If the distribution did not work out in that way, then the hypotheses would not be supported.

As might be supposed with all these data, the results were analyzed by a computer. The results of that portion of the data were combined with the results of other portions (the psychodynamic descriptions of the psychoanalytic clinical interviewers), and we then came to our findings.

Results

1. No cases of suicide were found among the accident victims.

2. The single issue in which accident victims were closer to suicide victims than to the appendectomy group was in alcohol intake. Table 1 (p. 97) summarizes some pertinent findings in regard to alcohol. The following points may be made in regard to the data shown in Table 1. Heavy daily drinking was noted in about one-fourth of both the appendectomy and suicide attempt sample, but of the subjects in the accident group, fully three-fourths indulged in heavy daily drinking. Increases in drinking were noted in a 6-mo. period in a small number of both accident (14 percent) and suicide (22 percent) subjects. *No* appendectomy subjects were considered to have increased their drinking in this period. In the 2 days prior to hospitali-

zation, 20% of accident subjects and 35% of suicide subjects increased their drinking, and again *no* appendectomy subjects did so.

3. Except for the alcohol hypothesis, none of the other suicidal and self-destructive hypotheses were supported. Although specifics varied with the nature of the particular hypothesis, the aim of the evaluation of each hypothesis was the same. That was to determine whether the accident victims (in the particular dimension of that hypothesis) were more like the suicide group or more like the appendectomy group. The picture presented by both the accident and appendectomy groups was close to what might be thought of as normal behavior (again, with the single exception of the alcohol hypothesis), whereas the suicide attempt group demonstrated depressive, impulsive , self-destructive behavior in a number of ways.

Discussion

First, some comment on the findings regarding drinking in our study. They replicate what has been found in many studies on accident, namely, that high drinking is correlated with automobile accident. Past work, however, leaves an unresolved issue in regard to the increased drinking. Is the accident the result of poor sensorimotor control because of physiological impairment, or is it linked to an increased state of tension of which drinking is an additional manifestation?

The increased drinking in 2-day and 6-mo. periods prior to hospitalization seen in both accident and suicide groups suggests that an increasing state of tension is operating in at least 20 percent of the accident group. The additional suggestion is that a higher percentage of accidents is correlated to something besides increasing tension. Twenty percent of accident victims showed increased drinking, but 76 percent of the accident group (as compared to 24 percent of the appendectomy group) showed daily drinking. The higher drinking rate in the accident victims may produce an impaired driving response or could also indicate an additional "psychological stress" factor.

What of the striking finding that there were almost no suicidal or self-destructive trends in our group of accident victims? First, let me reiterate that we specifically chose drivers of one-car accidents in order to maximize the possibility of finding such trends. Although it is possible that isolated cases or small groups of suicidal or self-destructive drivers exist, if our study was well done, the indication is that suicidal and self-destructive factors which we tested for do *not* play a significant role in the general accident picture.

In discussing this, some attention should be paid to the possible tendency that all or many psychoanalysts and psychotherapists have to project their own internal hypotheses and biases onto the situations, including their clinical material, with which they come into contact.

Many psychoanalysts have hypothesized self-destructive trends. They include Freud (*Beyond the Pleasure Principle*) and Karl Menninger (*Man Against Himself*). The possibility of a death instinct or other self-destructive factors producing such situations was theoretically sound. Moreover, a number of analysts, including my co-workers and myself, have postulated such trends. In fact, the hypotheses upon which the present study was based came from a series of previous psychoanalytic investigations. We fully expected to find at least some of these hypotheses borne out in the present study. Yet this did not occur.

It may be that suicide and psychological self-destruction are projected into the situation of accident partially because of previous thinking along this line and partially because of strict superego constellations in analysts. It may be that such self-destructive trends actually exist. But if they do, our study would suggest that if they occur, it is in other populations than that which we studied.

Some years ago, Hirshfield and Behan did a psychiatric study of industrial accidents. They found a high correlation with psychological factors of a self-destructive nature. However, they were dealing with a group of individuals who were different from the modal group of one-car accident drivers. Their group consisted of elderly people who were on the verge of being retired from their jobs and were facing various problems of old age and retirement. Under such circumstances, there may be a greater possibility of self-destruction in accident.

As a final point, I would like to comment on the theory of suicidal and self-destructive subselves. A number of psychological and psychoanalytic writers[11, 12] have postulated that under special life circumstances, special groups of characteristics come to the fore. Thus a person may be living a relatively non-self-destructive-life, but upon the occasion of a sudden and severe loss, a suicidal subself (based, perhaps, upon an identification with a suicidal parent) may become operative.

It may be similarly postulated that self-destructive characteristics tending toward the production of an automobile accident may be an important factor in the production of automobile accidents. Yet such subselves may be operative for only a short period of time so that when an accident victim is interviewed 1 to 3 wk. after his accident, evidence is not present for this subself. It may be replaced by another subself that has moved into ascendancy. From another standpoint, it may be that a need for

Table 1. *Alcoholic History of the Research Subjects (in percentages)*

Item	Accident	Suicide Attempt	Appendectomy
Heavy daily drinking	76*	30	24
Drinking increased in the 2 days prior to accident, suicide attempt, or appendectomy	20†	35‡	0
Drinking increased in the 6 mo. prior to accident, suicide attempt, or appendectomy	14	22	0

Chi-square comparisons between groups above resulted in the following statistically significant differences (at 0.02 level):
*Greater for accident than either suicide or appendectomy.
†Greater for accident than appendectomy.
‡Greater for suicide than appendectomy.

punishment has been satisfied by the resluts of the accident and this has led to a recession of the self-destructive subself.

Such an explanation could leave us with the possibility that many accident victims are self-destructive at the time of their accident but that evidence for it cannot later be found. This situation would pose an important problem for researchers into the psychology of automobile accident.

References

1. Tabachnick, N.: The psychology of fatal accident. in: Shneidman, E. (Ed.): Essays in Self-Destruction. New York, Science House, 1967.
2. Litman, R. E., and Tabachnick, N.: Fatal one-car accidents. Psychoanal. Quart 36:248–259, 1967.
3. Ford, R. and Moseley, A. L.: Motor vehicular suicides. In: *Research on Fatal Highway Collisions.* Cambridge, Mass., Harvard Medical School, 1961–1962.
4. Tabachnick, N., Litman, R. E., Osman, M., Jones, W., Cohn, J., Kasper, A., and Moffat, J.: Comparative psychiatric study of accidental and suicidal death. Arch. Gen. Psychiat. (Chicago) 14:60–68, 1966.
5. Moseley, A. L.: Research on Fatal Highway Collisions. Cambridge, Mass., Harvard Medical School, 1962–1963.
6. MacDonald, J. M.: Suicide and homicide by automobile. Amer. J. Psychiat. 4:366–370, 1964.
7. McCarroll, J. R., and Haddon, W.: A controlled study of fatal automobile accidents in New York City. J. Chronic Dis. 15:811–826, 1962.
8. Osman, M. P.: A psychoanalytic study of auto accident victims. Contemp. Psychoanal. 5:62–84, 1968.

9. Tabachnick, N., and Litman, R. E.: Character and life circumstance in fatal accident. Psychoanal. Forum 1:66–74, 1966.
10. Tabachnick, N.: The psychoanalyst as accident investigator. Behav. Res. Highway Safety 1:19–25, 1970.
11. Murray, H. A.: What should psychologists do about psychoanalysis? J. Abnorm. Soc. Psychol. 35:150, 1940.
12. Litman, R. E., and Tabachnick, N.: Psychoanalytic theories of suicide. In: Resnik, H. (Ed.): Suicidal Behaviors. New York, Little, Brown and Co., 1968.

Discussion by Paul Chodoff, M.D.

For a number of years, Dr. Tabachnik and his associates have been studying one of Freud's earliest and most firmly held ideas, that accidents and that even some examples of human self-injury are not really accidental, but are at least half-intentional; that men may harm themselves half-deliberately, against all reason and all self-preservative instincts. The particular example of a semipurposive self-injury they have concentrated on is the automobile accident, and they have chosen as their research strategy to compare and contrast these with suicides and suicidal attempts. In their investigations they have employed what they describe as psychoanalytic methods, and although I may have reservations about this statement, I have only praise for their attempt to bring into the public domain and subject to scientific scrutiny methods and conclusions sometimes wrongly held to exist in an island closed off from any extrapsychoanalytic scrutiny. The present paper is an effort to apply a combination of scientific rigor and psychoanalytic methods to the testing and documentation of formulations derived from the group's previous studies. The negative results which we have heard today call into question this previous work, and by allowing us to hear these results, Dr. Tabachnick has courageously presented a paper which is actually more interesting than the pious reaffirmations of previously held beliefs which too often pass for investigation in the field of psychoanalysis.

The previous papers alluded to but not described by Dr. Tabachnick and which provide the main source of the hypotheses tested in today's presentation consist of a comparison, by the method of psychological autopsy, of 15 suicides and 15 fatal accidents, and of interviews conducted by psychoanalysts with the survivors of nonfatal automobile accidents. Psychodynamic formulations and personality descriptions were derived from this material and elaborated in psychoanalytic terms. In general, both differences and similarities between the two groups were found but it was my impression after reading the papers that the differences were more striking than the similarities. Unlike suicidal and depressed persons, victims of the nonfatal automobile accidents were found to be basically action-oriented individuals with high self-esteem who regressed to infantile modes of impulse activity for ego restitutive purposes when faced with the stress of uncertain situations. Rather than seeking death these people were said to be seeking a new and better way to live, a picture quite different from that characteristic of most suicidal and depressed people. In view of this finding, I am puzzled and turn to Dr. Tabachnik for enlightenment as to why he and his co-workers expected the two groups to be much like others and framed their hypotheses to test the similarities between the accident victims and the suicide attempters.

Although I imagine Dr. Tabachnik made his paper general to avoid boring his audience with too many details, he leaves us in some ignorance about the compositions of the groups studied and the investigatory methods employed. He does not tell us how many subjects were in each group, whether he attempted matching, or whether any efforts were made to compensate for the fact that the investigators could not be blind to the group membership of the subjects interviewed. How did the psychoanalysts actually conduct their interviews? An average of 3 hr. per patient does not seem very long to bring about the kind of interpersonal trust and confidence which would allow for depth of psychological exploration, especially since the interviewer had to use the time to derive the answers to 205 questions. To state that psychoanalytic methods were used is, to my mind, not entirely accurate. Rather, the assumption was made that psychiatrists who had had psychoanalytic training would be more skilled in conducting fairly standard information-gathering interviews than nonpsychoanalysts. This is an important question because we have no assurance that the psychological resistance to which Dr. Tabachnick refers was overcome successfully in these interviews.

That many factors must combine fortuitously to culminate in an accident is of course obvious, and Dr. Tabachnick makes it clear that he is considering psychological factors only as one contributor to the end result. However, it is also true that if one has been involved in only a single serious automobile accident in his life the likelihood of psychological factors playing an important role would be considerably less than if one had established a pattern in which such accidents occurred repeatedly. Such a population would be difficult to get hold of, of course, since, for one thing, their life expectancy would not be very high; ideally, however, it would afford a better test of the hypotheses of the unconsciously motivated accident than the single-accident group. We enter here into the somewhat discredited notion of the accident-prone individual, and I agree that Dr. Tabachnick cannot be faulted for being unable to reconcile his experimental design with the stubborn refusal of human beings to behave like experimental animals. An experimental group of frequent traffic violations might provide interesting data on self-destructive tendencies, although they could only potentially be considered suicide attempters.

Other problems with the experimental design include the fact that although certain practical difficulties would have prevented the use of successful suicides as a control group, the clinical and personality characteristics of suicide attempters are known to differ significantly from those of the former. Also, the necessary elimination of accidents involving more than one driver deprives the investigators of a possibly significant group in whom intrapunitive factors might be combined with externally directed feelings of hostility and revenge.

The results of the investigation amount to a negation of the hypotheses that victims of serious accidents are more like suicide attempters than so-called normals, and affirmation of the well-established statistic that accidents are associated with drunkenness. The latter result is not surprising; the former is, since I venture to suggest that most analysts, including myself, would share the bias, as in Dr. Wold's paper, that unconscious motivational factors of a self-destructive character play a significant role in at least some accidents. However, the entirely negative results of this study must be somewhat puzzling even to those who accept alcoholism as a sufficient cause of automobile accidents since it is strange that the accident group should be relatively normal psychologically according to the criteria employed unless one also accepts the unlikely hypothesis that there are no psychological abnormalities in alcoholics. Of course, this apparent discrepancy can be explained at least partially if it is postulated that the psychopathological patterns of alcoholics differ so significantly from those of depressed persons and accident victims that they were not tapped in the 12 hypotheses tested in the study. Such an explanation, however, would contravene another generally accepted belief among psychiatrists and psychoanalysts that alcoholism is one of the ways in which the seeds of self-destructiveness manifest themselves. I would suggest that further studies of the psychology of accident victims might include a control group of alcoholics without histories of severe accidents to see if they differ significantly from alcoholics who do have serious accident histories.

Finally, if we believe that both accidents and alcoholism represent modes of acting out of inherent self-destructive tendencies, how can we account for the negative results of Dr. Tabachnick's investigation? I do not find myself persuaded by his suggestion that the accident behavior is due to the temporary ascendancy of a putative self-destructive subself which can fade into repression once its needs have been met since this explanation would not account for the absence in the study group of a number of long-term stable personality characteristics of an aberrant nature which are included in the hypotheses tested. My review of this paper and the previous work of Dr. Tabachnick's group suggests three possible explanations. First, the investigators, although psychoanalytically trained, did not have sufficient contact over a sufficiently long period of time to penetrate the psychological resistance with which they were faced. Second, I do not believe that single-accident victims constitute an adequate experimental group in view of the multiplicity of the factors which can enter into the production of a particular automobile accident. Third, I question the framing of the hypotheses to maximize the similarities between the accident group and individuals whose self-destructive tendencies manifest themselves in depressive illness and suicide attempts when these similarities may be overshadowed by conspicuous differences between the two groups.

Schizophrenia as Conflict and Defense: Implications for Therapy and Research

JACK L. RUBINS, M.D.

Until now, the psychoanalytic approach to the schizophrenias—both in theory and in therapeutic techniques—has been most variable and inconclusive. Published reports have indicated results ranging from most successful to failure, from excessive optimism to undeserved nihilism. Relatively few analysts have described their techniques and therapeutic results in much detail. Too often there is a vagueness or imprecision about the pathological condition, the concepts used to define it, the type of patient, and the therapeutic interactions. In this paper I shall attempt to outline a new holistic psychoanalytic view of the schizophrenic process, briefly describe some of its implications for therapy, and then present an ongoing clinical research program in which principles and methods are being clarified and their effectiveness is being tested and evaluated.

While treating schizophrenic patients in private practice over the past 20 yr., I have been impressed by the great importance of their emotional and attitudinal conflicts. In fact I have come to feel that conflict is the major dynamic psychopathological phenomenon in these conditions.

That such conflict can produce abnormal psychic states is not a new or original concept. Masserman[1] has shown that conflict can give rise to neuroses, alcoholism, and psychotic-type symptoms in animals, but the danger of extrapolating from animals to human beings must of course be considered. Within the Freudian theories, neurotic symptoms were ascribed to conflicts between libidinal and ego-restrictive forces. According to Horney, dynamic conflicts between any contradictory but compulsive attitudes were held responsible for neurotic development.

The etiological role of conflict in schizophrenia has also been previously noted, for instance in Bleuler's concept of ambivalence as a primary symptom. However, this notion implied more a static condition of contradictory attitudes rather than dynamically active opposing forces. It was also considered in the classical psychoanalytic view of the psychoses as exemplified both in the conflict between libidinal and aggressive drives and in the theory of ego splitting by ambivalent introjected objects. But the application of these concepts has been limited by the questionable presence and action of such supposedly instinctual drives as well as by the purely cognitive nature of inner object representations, so that their dynamic effects cannot be followed to their fullest clinical application. Recently, using the Sullivanian approach, several authors have emphasized the importance of interpersonal conflicts in the schizophrenic's relationships. Schacht and Kempster,[2] Burnham,[3] and Stierlin[4] mention such conflicts as needing to be manipulative versus needing to be praised, needing to control versus needing to be controlled, needs for integration versus differentiation, for stabilization versus stimulation, for sameness versus difference, for closeness versus distance, for gratification versus frustration. They feel that the major goal of therapy is to reconcile such conflicting attitudes.

Following the dynamic-holistic concepts of Horney, modified so as to be applicable to the psychoses, I have described the psychogenesis and development of schizophrenia, the psychodynamics of its clinical symptoms, and a therapeutic approach.[5-7] Since most of these notions go beyond the scope of this chapter, I shall limit myself here to the recapitulation of those related to the nature and role of conflict.

I believe that the schizophrenia process is a pathological form and direction of development which need not manifest itself in "typical" psychotic symptoms. It has similarities to as well as differences from the neurotic form of growth. This process can be divided into three parts: prepsychotic development, psychosis itself, and the process of reversal of psychosis. Prepsychotic development is initiated in the child in reaction to definable conscious or unconscious attitudes of parents, and it may be maintained by continued interaction with such attitudes. The resulting personality disturbance encompasses two aspects of the child's growth pattern.

First, *maturational development* is distorted. This would normally include formation of a body image, its inclusion into a reasonable self-concept, and then transformation of this into an accepted identity (identity formation). This process is constant and ongoing throughout life and is normally harmonious and sequential although varying in rate at different periods. It is vulnerable to psychotogenic influences, more so at special times such as adolescence. Any aspect of this tristage development may be adversely affected, and by many internal or external factors. These may include constitutional or psychobiological ones like organ defects, rapid body changes due to growth, chemical or enzymatic dysfunctions, impaired psychological capacity for filtering external stimuli, lowered tolerance for anxiety, excessive need intensity, etc. Or distortion of maturational development may result from social factors like parental rejection of special aspects of the child, poor physical or emotional contact with parents, cultural influences, peer pressures, etc. Specific distortions of this process, such as impaired body image, irrational self-concept, or poor identity formation, can predispose to specific symptoms.

Second, *emotional development* is also distorted. Normally this would be characterized by adoption of specific needs, attitudes, and behavior toward parents so as to provide the child with the optimal love, acceptance, and security possible. Following Horney's schema, these might consist of compliance or dependence, assertiveness or aggressivity, and detachment or withdrawal. In a healthy home atmosphere, these can be freely expressed, appropriately and to a normal degree. But faced with pathological parental attitudes, these infantile interpersonal attitudes become compulsive since they are motivated by fear of rejection, loss of love, and potential hostility if not actual separation ("basic infantile anxiety"). Any attitudes contrary to the socially needed expressed ones must be repressed, but they remain dynamically active from within, producing partly conscious, partly unconscious conflicts. When this parental milieu is also unstable, inconsistent, intangible, yet repressive, these reactive attitudes of the child become more volatile and intense but less able to provide stabilization or gratification. As a result, the anxiety and conflict is also more intense and becomes preschizophrenic rather than normal or neurotic. It then requires further defensive measures.

The utilization of secondary defensive maneuvers to avoid both this anxiety/conflict and the maturational impairment now constitutes the further prepsychotic development. It is now self-perpetuated, intrapsychic as much as interpersonal, and against the attitudes of others. The defensive measures can include an intensification of the original orientation (pathological dependence or other-directedness, aggressiveness or domination, isolation), and a pathological self-aggrandizement, expressed in grandiosity, extreme arrogance, excessive narcissism, or obsessive perfectionism. Each of these tendencies will be accompanied by corresponding exaggerated needs, demands on others (claims), pressures on the self (shoulds), and inhibitions. All such traits are highly invested with pride, therefore unstable and vulnerable to being disproved or contradicted. They render the person hypersensitive to hurt or frustration. Such hurt pride can produce, in turn, intense self-hate or self-contempt with all its concomitant feelings: inadequacy, humiliation, worthlessness, ugliness, loathesomeness, etc. In the prepsychotic state these latter attitudes toward self are often intensified by coexisting feelings of being defective owing to the maturational impairment. This type of reactive feeling, so often occurring in the schizophrenic, necessitates unconscious attempts to restore the exaggerated and irrational pride. These often consist of the violent rage or vindictive outbursts so typical of many psychotics.

Additional conflict can be generated by the added contradiction between the grandiose and despised self-image which the prepsychotic and psychotic feels himself to be. More stringent defensive measures are then needed to avoid this increased sense of conflict, even of chaos. These may include stilling all change or activity, whether internal (sensations, emotions) or external (changes in space, time, sequence, or position, new situations or relationships); the direct benumbing of feelings or inner experiences (alienation from self); living an imitative or "as-if" life; externalizing inner experiences or living through others; excessive fantasy life or mechanical intellectualizing; concretization of thought processes; and avoidance of situations or relationships in which intense conflicting attitudes or emotions may be aroused.

So long as these characterological defensive measures can more or less successfully cope with the underlying conflict, even with some anxiety, the person remains a prepsychotic character disorder or a latent (non-psychotic) schizophrenic or a borderline condition. But if either the inner conflicts or the maturational impairment is exacerbated, threatening the effectiveness of any of these defensive maneuvers, then the psychosis itself can be precipitated. In such a case, the defensive measure itself may become the typical schizophrenic symptom. Such triggering can occur either spontaneously owing to the emergence into awareness of some partly unconscious attitude, or from the impact of a stressful external event.

To summarize, this view postulates that schizophrenia is wholly defensive against the conflict of compulsive emotions or attitudes, both interpersonal and intrapsychic, in active dynamic opposition. It disagrees with the concept of this psychosis as a "collapse" of defenses with subsequent regression. This includes the several definitions of regression: the classical one, return to a state of "normal" infantile narcissism and omnipotence and to an unformed, undifferentiated ego, with primary process thinking; the Jacksonian one, return to a more primitive, archaic form of functioning; and Fairburn's definition, return to a state of dependency. Rather than being simpler and more primitive, the symptom is seen as more complex, expressing many levels of meaning or communication at once. Each symptom is related to definable dynamic conflicts; any intellectual disturbance is secondary to the emotional process.

Several implications for therapy flow from this approach. Since these have been presented elsewhere in detail, they will only be sketched schematically here. First, the contributory role of organic factors in the etiology of schizophrenia is accepted, insofar as they modify the maturational process. These make up the substratum on which the emotional disturbance impinges. Therefore, the therapeutic use of drugs or biosocial methods (reduction of external stimuli, structuring the milieu, etc.) can be acceptably combined with psychoanalysis as part of total therapy. But they remain ancillary rather than primary, intended either to repair the maturational defect or to facilitate analytic work. When such drugs, for instance, are used, attention must be paid to their extrinsic dynamic significance for the patient along with their intrinsic pharmacological effects.

Second, psychoanalytic therapy, suitably modified for the individual patient, can be used to reverse the schizophrenic process. During such therapy there will occur a constant shifting of the patient's personality traits, emotions, experiences, and attitudes toward himself and others. These always exist in a functional rather than static organization, according to the constellation of conflicts and defensive measures noted above. Each attribute has a peremptory force and is in dynamic relation with other emotional traits. Each can thus reinforce, inhibit, modify, or conflict with other attributes. This occurs out of awareness, but each can emerge into consciousness; it will then demand satisfaction, produce needs or strivings, or press toward action. Any attribute will be experienced in a positive way to the extent that it is in keeping with the irrationally glorified self-image. Or it will be defended against to the extent that it is unfavorable and unacceptable to this self-image, therefore emotionally painful and threatening. Any attribute may thus be valued and admired or hated and despised, whether experienced in one's own self or seen in others. It will then be identified with as part of self and as subject, or as other than self and as the object of experience.

The analytic process consists of such personality changes and psychic movements over varying periods of time, in observable and definable patterns. Although their superficial manifestations—psychotic symptoms, overt behaviors, specific preoccupations, disturbed areas of social functioning—may change and seem to become significant at different moments, these are of lesser importance to the analyst than the underlying dynamic movements and process. Such symptoms are nonspecific in the sense that different conflicts or defensive solutions may produce the same symptom, or any one attitude emerging into awareness may give rise to differing symptoms. If the basal causal conflicts can be influenced by therapeutic activity, the resulting symptomatic expression will disappear.

Third, every communication during analytic therapy, whether expressed by action, nonverbal means, interpersonal attitude, or verbal statement, can express one or several simultaneous levels of unconscious feeling or thought. The mode of expression can also vary, so that the unconscious experience can give rise to another thought, feeling, action, image, or somatic symptoms. As a result, there may be much change in symptoms with little basic dynamic movement, or little symptomatic improvement with much real underlying change. The analyst must be constantly aware of this ever-changing configuration and alert to whatever emotion may be emerging at the moment. Therapeutic progress can be produced by directing the patient's attention to that attitude, feeling, cognitive meaning, or other expression the analyst deems most meaningful. The most productive of progress will be that most available for thoughtful work and most acceptable to the patient's total defensive state, in the sense of provoking least anxiety or emotional pain and most awareness. Its context can vary from the totally concrete and situational, to the emotional reaction to an external event, to a more totally intrapsychic or unconscious level.

Fourth, using flexible technique parameters, the creation of a viable doctor-patient relationship is a primary and often most difficult requirement of therapy. This must take into account the patient's intensely demanding and conflicting needs and interpersonal attitudes. He is fearful of intimate emotional contact which would cause him to experience the conflict between his compliance-dependency needs and his dominating-manipulative needs, as well as his inner impairment. He must retain a certain distance. Yet he simultaneously needs closeness to avoid experiencing his loneliness, emptiness, and self-contempt. He vacillates between these two extremes, feeling anxiety and even nonexistence if he goes too far in either direction. He also seeks stable external objects and other persons to offset his inner shifting and provide consistent limits and boundaries. Yet he resents any awareness of this need, which is often experienced as external coercion or restriction. He expects and demands to be treated by the analyst with unconditional love, gratification, recognition, and uniqueness, to be given power and freedom, all in keeping with his grandiose self-image of which he is unaware. At the same time he usually experiences only his despised self, his self-loathing, his worthlessness, inadequacy, and sickness; he anticipates being scorned by the analyst. As he shifts between these poles, the analyst likewise becomes either idealized and loved or despised and hated.

The optimal kind of active intervention from the analyst would consist of wholehearted emotional engagement. This refers to involvement in the emotional experiences of the patient, the feeling of care and concern and hope and acceptance for the patient rather than only detached interest.

Fifth, the resolution of the many conflicts can be induced by several kinds of activities by the analyst, which I would consider interpretative in the broadest sense of the term. These might include noncognitive interpretations, intended to provide support, encouragement, interest, stimulation, or simply human presence; experience-intensifying interpretations to call attention to inner happenings as immediate sensate experience, needed to reform or strengthen identity and decrease emotional alienation from self; cognitive interpretations to define attitudes in conflict and show how they are intense, irrational, pervasive of the personality, entering into behavior, and destructive; disillusioning interpretations aimed at undermining the deeper, pride-invested dynamic feelings about self which underlie the conflictive attitudes; reality corrective interpretations to provide alternative explanations of psychotic distortions; and growth-promoting interpretations to strengthen self-esteem and give direction to constructive strivings.

Even though this holistic-dynamic approach has proven effective in a relatively small number of schizophrenic patients treated in private analytic practice by a few analysts, including myself, I have felt it essential to test its efficacy further by clinical research. There are many reasons why such research is needed. For one, the usefulness of psychoanalytic therapy for schizophrenia is being questioned in today's psychiatric climate. The community mental health movement, spurred by the demands for therapy of the hitherto neglected lower economic population, has been emphasizing treatment of the greatest number of persons, with rapid and super-ficial improvement rather than the slower and deeper but more lasting personality change. This has directed attention toward such forms of intervention as behavior therapy, group or encounter therapy, drug therapy, or direct environmental manipulation. Unfortunately, the results of these therapies of expediency, of quantity rather than quality, leave much to be desired in many cases. Even though manifest symptoms can be ameliorated by these forms of treatment and the patient becomes somewhat better able to "adjust" socially, covert impairments may continue to incapacitate him. According to Mosher,[8] only 20 to 30 percent of such patients can function even at a low-average level, in even relatively nondemanding situations. Many then spend their life in loneliness or isolation, or in barren, routine activity, or functioning in a mechanical, joyless way far below their real social, intellectual, and emotional level, often feeling emptiness, "quiet desperation," and apprehension. The destructive effects and suffering inflicted by such patients on families or others with whom they come into contact are incalculable. Another aspect is the continued, prolonged (often lifelong) need for medication, with its possible side effects or decreas-ing effectiveness, and need for constant medical supervision. Still another is the rate of relapse. It has been estimated that nationwide, 50 percent of first-hospitalization acute schizophrenics undergo a second episode within 2 yr. Certainly all acute schizophrenics cannot use, accept, or respond to intensive psychoanalytic therapy. In our own program, perhaps a third of the applicants are suitable, given the limitations of our physical facilities and staff; this could be increased somewhat if our means were improved. Nevertheless it is incumbent upon those of us who are concerned about this unhappy state of affairs to reevaluate this claimed role of psychoanalysis, to seek ways and means of testing, improving, and extending its applicability to the psychoses.

Another reason is that even many analysts have been reluctant to treat the schizophrenias. For some, this hesitation is a carry-over from Freud's position that psychotics "become inaccessible to the influence of psychoanalysis and cannot be cured by our efforts."[9] Others have been deterred by practical difficulties of therapy either inherent in the theoretical framework or characteristic of the psychoses themselves. These have in-cluded the pessimistic view of an inevitably poor prognosis and expectation of poor therapeutic results; the presence of supposedly unchangeable genetic, constitutional, or organic factors; the long time required for treatment; the problem of handling the intense emotional swings, or their opposite, the lack of emotionality; the problem of dealing with impulsive-ness, aggressiveness, or acting out; the difficulty in making a "positive" therapeutic relationship; the intense, seemingly insatiable demands on the therapist; the difficulty in communicating or understanding some patients; the belief that unconscious content cannot be interpreted because of the alleged collapse of defenses; and the need to lead the patient back from the supposed regressed "infantile state" by having to provide "oral supplies" to make up for former deprivation. And this reluctance has persisted in spite of the fact that more schizophrenics are now appearing in analysts' offices under newer official policies favoring ambulatory rather than in-hospital treatment. It is therefore necessary to dissipate such negative attitudes held by so many analysts by providing evidence, if possible, to the contrary.

A third reason is that most previously published reports of analytic therapy have been anecdotal and dealt with 1 or very few patients. I do not decry the importance of the single clinical case report. It can give considerable and valuable information, and much of our great progress in the field has resulted from such studies. Also, the anecdotal description may be the most valid and appropriate for describing such complex on-going situations as the therapeutic one, where processes, movements, interactions, and dynamic concepts must be depicted. On the other hand, the anecdotal description, however sensitive and perceptive the observing analyst, is still valid only within the limiting framework of the preexisting assumptions held. It is thus subject to the unwitting bias of the observer. This could involve such variables as the subjective equation of the therapist himself, the introduction of inferable along with observable factors, the possible blind spots of the observer, the finding of observations tending to validate the previous theoretical bases thereby creating a self-fulfilling prophesy, and the role of wish fulfillment in evaluating positive results. I believe that the anecdotal clinical case study and the modern research approach need not be mutually exclusive if the latter is considered simply a process of *describing* functional parts of the whole with precision, rather than a reductionistic means of *explaining* the whole through isolated parts. In modern research terms, the case study would be considered a "backward" or retrospective type and its major value would be preliminary, to show the possibilities of a therapeutic tool. It would have to be applied then to "forward" or predictive studies which can test the value and effects of the tool on other cases.

Related to this point, previous published results of analysis of schizo-phrenics have been variable. Most reported case studies by individual analysts, regardless of the theoretical approach used, have claimed significant improvements in the patients described. These have included traditional as well as modified Freudian methods. Among these might be mentioned the early ego-analytic and ego-strengthening "encapsulation" techniques of analysts like Bychowski,[10] Federn,[11] Alexander,[12] and Schilder[13]; the "symbolic realization" of Sechehaye[14]; the maternal-replacement approach of Schwing[15] and its later variant, the "objects relations" therapy of Azima[16]; the "direct analysis" of Rosen[17]; the superego (father) replacement technique of Wechsler[18]; the classical method of Boyer[19] using few technique parameters; and the broadly modified "modern psychoanalysis" of Spotnitz.[20] Several European analysts have advocated an eclectic approach, combining aspects of all these methods.[21-23] Going beyond the classical theories and focusing on the patient's distorted interpersonal relationships, positive results have been reported by such analysts as Sullivan,[24] Fromm-Reichmann,[25] Powder-maker,[26] Searles,[27] and Will.[28] Arieti has combined this approach with a concomitant emphasis on the primary-process thought disorder, the "formal psychotic defense mechanisms," and creative potentials in psychotic reintegration.[29] Application of the Horney approach has also reportedly produced positive results for Kilpatrick,[30] Metzger,[31] Hott,[32] Boigon,[33] and Sheiner,[34] as well as my own results (which have been mixed).

Recent larger-scale research studies on the effects of modified psychoanalytic therapies on chronic hospitalized schizophrenics have shown equivocal effects. In one such project,[35] those patients receiving "active" or "ego" psychoanalysis (nonspecific in its theoretical framework) were discharged sooner than those without it and showed a more balanced general positive change. But those with medication showed a greater improvement in specific target symptoms than those not receiving it. In two other studies[36,37] the patients on analytically oriented psychotherapy showed no better evidence of "positive outcome" than patients on drugs alone, but a year after discharge, the therapy group showed a greater number of positive personality changes. Of course, these latter projects were carried out in different settings and different-type patients—chronic and hospitalized—than the other case reports. Nevertheless, the almost uniformly good results reported for such different forms of analytic therapy, as well as the success of any one form in the hands of one analyst and its lack of success when used by another analyst, raise serious questions. To what extent are such positive results coincidental or idiosyncratic to the particular analyst rather than due to any particular theoretical framework, technique, or setting? It is therefore essential to define concepts precisely and clarify therapeutic operations by further clinical research so as to permit validation and replication by others.

One final reason for research is that most of these reports of psychoanalytic results are in terms of symptomatic improvement, i.e., amelioration of acute psychotic behavior, discharge from hospital, or ability to function socially at a minimal level. With some exceptions, the degree and form of personality change, the level of function in terms of the patient's optimal capacities, and the long-term outcome in terms of recurrence or rehospitalization are seldom indicated. A few authors do refer to resolution of the "psychotic core" but this is vague, and some indicate that long-term psychoanalysis of the standard type is required after the acute condition is relieved. It is therefore necessary to develop therapeutic goals and evaluative measures of long-term effectiveness and outcome which will be fair to the method of therapy used—in our case to the holistic-dynamic, conflict-resolving, and growth-directed form of psychoanalysis. These must include criteria for involvement and changeful progress in analysis, for personality change, and for constructive growth in terms of optimal patient potentials (self-realization). Although this latter factor has long been an integral aspect of this analytic approach, it is only recently that it is being recognized by other analytic therapists, as Mosher has emphasized.[8]

With these considerations in mind, 3 yr. ago we set up an analytically oriented day-center program for acute schizophrenic patients on a trial basis. Here we have been treating 20 patients between 18 and 30 yr. old, who no longer require full-time hospitalization but whose psychotic symptoms are still too disturbing to permit them to function in their habitual activities. "Acute" refers to the relatively rapid onset of psychotic symptoms within 5 yr. before coming to us, regardless of the number of hospitalizations during this time. This would probably correspond to the "reactive" rather than the "process" form of schizophrenia. Severity of symptoms and subform of the psychosis are not considered significant. The patients receive milieu therapy, group therapy, drug therapy when necessary, and individual psychoanalytic therapy on a twice- or three-session-per-week basis. There are eight treating analysts, half being certified analysts, half being candidates-in-training under close clinical supervision. The average patient stay has been thus far about 2 yr. Since this situation approaches private practice conditions in that the patients are free agents, suitability for the program requires availability for long-term therapy, namely a voluntary acceptance of regular attendance for an indefinite period. It also requires some positive motivation for therapy other than the need for symptom relief alone; this means at least a willingness for self-exploration and a desire for personality change and fuller living.

During these preliminary years, the therapeutic results obtained for a significant percentage and number of patients have been encouraging. These have consisted mainly of improved interpersonal relations (with family, friends, sexual partners, social-vocational rehabilitation (return to school or work where this had been previously impossible), better organization of self and perception of reality, raising of the functional intellectual level, and lessening of the acute psychotic symptoms (delusions, hallucinations, etc.). For most patients, such improvements have tended to be fluctuating. They have been evaluated generally through independent clinical observation, although in some cases by repeated psychological testing as well. We feel that this is too short an elapsed time to assess or to expect fundamental personality change through the analytic work. However, we now believe that these results justify setting up a more structured and detailed research project intended to formally evaluate the therapeutic improvement and to compare the relative effectiveness of the analytic therapy with each of the other therapeutic modalities in the comprehensive program.

In this final section of my chapter I wish to present some of the implications of our therapeutic approach for future research, derived from our past experiences, which we have had to deal with. I shall pass over those problems having to do with research in intensive psychotherapy in general; these involve broad philosophical and methodological questions which would take me beyond the scope of this paper. These are issues like the morality of using patients for experimental study, whether the clinical psychoanalyst is qualified for and can do good research, whether the research procedures and settings negate the basic therapeutic process or goals, and whether the isolation and measurement of specific variables constitute an artificial fragmentation, mechanization, or reductionism which does injustice to the essential human subjectivity and wholeness. A spate of recently published articles and books[38-41] have well discussed these questions, and Strupp and Bergin[42] have summarized them in an excellent review. I shall limit myself only to the psychoanalytic therapy of the schizophrenias and to the use of our holistic approach in particular.

One first implication of such an investigation relates to its methodology and puts into question the very need for further formal research. If it is to test the effectiveness of our approach—or of any psychoanalytic method— it must be evaluated against suitable *controls*. This requires the selection of a group of patients as similar as possible (according to standardized criteria like age, economic level, type of onset, intellectual level, etc.) to those in psychoanalytic therapy, who will not receive this therapy and who will be similarly evaluated over the same intervals. Our projected plan will involve comparison control groups since several therapeutic modalities are being used in the comprehensive program. Each group will receive one type of therapy, i.e., psychoanalysis alone, drug therapy alone, milieu therapy (day care) alone, the full comprehensive program (all therapies combined), or no treatment. We recognize that in a strict sense, a true no-treatment state is impossible since external events will exert a therapeutic effect, for better or worse, nonetheless. We plan simply to enroll the patient in the project after initial screening and then only see him at infrequent but regular intervals, without any formal psychotherapy or drugs prescribed (except in case of real emergency). As an additional comparison measure, we plan similarly to evaluate a group of nonpsychotic (psychoneurotic) patients being treated by the same analysts. Although I have emphasized the great significance of the subjective equation of the analyst in influencing progress and outcome, it is necessary to obviate this influence—or at least to equalize it across the different groups of patients. Therefore, in this first phase of evaluation of effectiveness of psychoanalytic therapy as a whole, each analyst will be assigned a patient from the five groups.

Another implication is that the selected variables for evaluation of change must have relevance to the psychodynamic process as well as to symptomatic manifestations. Since in this view of schizophrenia, the ongoing dynamic process is primary and the symptoms express transitory defensive reactions, therapy must also be directed at that underlying process with the immediate behavior considered of secondary importance. This concept has proven most difficult for the staff (including the treating analysts) to grasp, to accept, and to apply therapeutically. In effect, it involves the use of psychoanalytic principles for the psychoses, i.e., verbal expression rather than "doing," concern with intrapsychic or interpersonal events rather than external situation, concern for the emotional and attitudinal rather than the concrete, and primary emphasis on long-term personality change rather than immediate changing happenings. This is significant both for setting therapeutic goals as well as for determining criteria for handling behavioral symptoms (as against the long-term personality changes). Certainly symptoms must be dealt with insofar as they can create problems in the patient-group relationships. But this is more relevant for the ongoing operation of the day-center facility (or hospital) rather than for the psychoanalysis itself. They are also significant to the extent that they can influence analytic progress; and the judicial use of the ancillary therapies like drugs, group influence, or occupational therapy can facilitate the analytic work when symptoms like excessive anxiety or agitation, depression or defensive concreteness are thereby lessened. By the same token, these ancillary therapies can also obstruct or modify the analytic situation.

However, in our experience until now, both the nonpsychiatric professional personnel and the psychoanalysts have tended to overemphasize the importance and gravity of each fluctuating symptom and each problem situation the patient brings in. It has been too often felt that each such situation had to be handled by direct control (excessive use of drugs, authoritarian direction, environmental manipulation, etc.) rather than by trying to resolve the underlying conflictual emotional motivations. This therapeutic attitude would seem to be related in part to the same factors, mentioned before, which contribute to the reluctance of many analysts to treat psychotics. In part it seems to result from a deep-seated, perhaps unconscious fear of schizophrenia, of the patient going "out of control," of aggressiveness, of the irreversibility of symptoms. In part it may reflect a certain need for the concrete, a need for action, an impatience or personal insecurity or overidentification with the patient's helplessness. In some instances, these attitudes have changed as the analyst became less apprehensive, more familiar with the type of patient, more experienced and more aware of the fluctuating, symbolic nature of the symptoms. Such attitudes would be partly related to the A-B therapist types described by Whitehorn and Betz,[43] which made for a differential success in treating neurotic versus psychotic patients.

These observations indicate that the evaluation of the effectiveness of any psychoanalytic therapy for schizophrenia will require the clearest possible definition of the operations and techniques employed by the analyst during the therapeutic transactions, even though general principles may have already been enunciated. In addition, the analyst's personality traits —feelings, attitudes toward himself and toward the patient, values, inhibitions—both conscious and unconscious, and particularly as they apply to the schizophrenic, must be given careful consideration in their effects on analytic progress. In our own project, these factors will be given appropriate concern in a second phase after we have assessed whether analysis itself compares with the other methods of therapy.

Another implication of our research is that with such a multitude of variables, manifest and unconscious, behavioral and dynamic, subtle and subjective, we have had to form groups of related variables into broader categories. We have therefore developed a schema for expectation of outcome, categorizing our ideal aims of analytic therapy (see Table 1).

Table 1. Expectation of Outcome as Categories of Dependent Variables

Behavioral-Symptom Correlates	Hoped-for Outcome	Category of Dependent Variables
(a) Hallucinations ⎫ Poor perception (b) Delusions ⎬ of reality, testing ⎪ of reality, relating ⎭ to reality	Disappearance	I. Psychotic symptoms
(c) Active conflict: Vacillation, indecision (choice making); Inertia (action) Uncertainty, ambivalence (ideas, values, feelings)	More decisiveness and certainty	
(d) Anxiety: free-floating; fixed (phobias, etc., psychophysiological symptoms)	Lessening, or greater tolerance for	
(e) Poor impulse control, acting out; intolerance for delay or frustration	Rational control; ability to postpone gratification; lesser intensity of needs.	
(f) Hypersensitivity to change (inner or external) Psychomotor and psychic retardation	Tolerance for change	
(g) Depersonalization phenomena; somatic delusions	Disappearance; more realistic, acceptable body-image, self-concept, identity	
(a) Illogical or disjointed associations	Logical thinking	II. Thought processes
(b) Concrete or personalized references	Greater capacity for abstract thinking	
(c) Inability to concentrate or focus thoughts	Ability to concentrate	
(a) Poor family relationships (with spouse, parents, children, siblings)	Improvement; more intimate, conflict-free relationships	III. Interpersonal-social relations
(b) Fear of taking future family role: marriage, having children, work, commitment, responsibility, etc.	Acceptance of normal family role consistent with age, status, etc.	
(c) Social withdrawal, isolation, lack of friends	Better relating to peers	
(d) Poor heterosexual relationships: Fear of sexual contacts, intimacy	Better heterosexual relating	

Table 1 (*Continued*)

Behavioral-Symptom Correlates	Hoped-for Outcome	Category of Dependent Variables
Poor sexual intercourse (anxiety-producing, detached, painful)	Enjoyable, emotionally fulfilling intercourse	
Incapacity for genuine love	Genuine love, tenderness	
Fear of emotional engagement	Emotional engagement, commitment	
Sexual dysfunctions (premature ejaculation, impotence, frigidity, dyspareunia)	Normal sexual function	
Compulsive sexual perversions (voyeurism, fetishism, exhibitionism, homosexuality)	Noncompulsive sexual activity	
(e) Uncertainty about vocation; inability to work; frequent job changes	Desire to work; enjoyable work activity; ability to hold job consistent with capacities	
(f) Compulsive (need-driven) expansive attitudes (domination, manipulative, exploitative, sadistic)	Noncompulsive assertiveness	
(g) Compulsive (need-driven) self-effacement (compliance, dependence, submissiveness, masochism)	Noncompulsive dependency	
(h) Irrational idealization (need satisfying) of others	Realistic view of others; healthy (non-need-driven) love	
(i) Vicarious living through others; overfocussing on externals; other-directedness	Self-directedness; concern with own interests; self-acceptance	
(a) Discrepancy between intellectual capacity and actual intellectual functioning (pseudoimpairment of IQ; scattering of performance)	Ability to function at real level of intelligence	IV. Intellectual functioning
(b) Learning blocks; inability to concentrate, to study, to absorb	Ability to learn	
(a) Lack of curiosity or interest in self	Curiosity, concern about self	V. Involvement in therapy
(b) Passivity; poor initiative;	Initiative, spontaneity,	

Table 1 (*Continued*)

Behavioral-Symptom Correlates	Hoped-for Outcome	Category of Dependent Variables
expecting other to do for him	activity	
(c) More attention to situation or to externals than to self	Greater attention to self	
(d) Excessive acting out; overemphasis on "doing"	Replacement of action by verbal or reflective activity	
(e) Lack of dynamic movement or change; sterile verbalizing	Appearance of movement	
(f) Remoteness from inner experiences; failure to apply awareness to self	Closening to inner experiences	
(g) Poor expression of, awareness of, and involvement in emotions	Freer emotionality, letting go, involvement in emotions	
(a) Irrational grandiosity (various specific aspects: power, goodness, righteousness, abilities, etc.)	Self-concept in keeping with real attributes and abilities	VI. Attitudes toward self (self evaluative; reduction of self-idealization)
(b) Irrational self-denigration (feelings of inadequacy, worthlessness, inferiority, self-dislike; guilt, self-blame)	Normal self-esteem; self-liking	
(c) Self-punitive, self-destructive behavior (accident proneness, suicidal trends, destructive habits, self-accusing, etc.)	Self-acceptance	
(d) Compulsively perfectionistic behavior	Greater flexibility; acceptance of imperfections; fewer demands on self	
(e) Irrational claims or entitlements (varying forms: expecting special treatment, love, admiration, attention, immunity, etc.)	Awareness of real limitations	
(f) Excessive narcissism (self-admiration, preoccupation with self, looks, etc.)	Acceptance of flaws; self-esteem in keeping with real self	
(a) Inability to make choices	Ability to choose, acceptance of consequences	VII. Autonomy and competence

Table 1 (*Continued*)

Behavioral-Symptom Correlates	Hoped-for Outcome	Category of Dependent Variables
(b) Inability to take responsibility	Acceptance of responsibility	
(c) Passivity, other-directedness	Self-directedness	
(d) Egocentricity; interest mainly in compulsive need satisfaction	Concern with genuine self-interest	
(e) Egocentric, selfish interest in others	Genuine concern for others; ability to give emotionally	
(f) Poor real self-esteem; excessive irrational pride	Healthier self-esteem; pride in real abilities	
(g) Benumbing, avoidance, lack of awareness of feelings	Greater awareness and involvement in feelings	
(h) Poor body image, self-concept, and identity	Clearer body image, self-concept; completer identity	
(i) Aimless, driven, nonproductive activity	More productive, less driven activity	
(j) Lack of satisfaction or enjoyment from activities	Satisfaction from activities, work	
(k) Lack of positive enjoyment	Capacity for positive enjoyment and contentment	
(l) Avoidance of normal unpleasant experiences, frustrations, conflicts of living	Willingness and ability to tolerate normal painful experiences	

These goals are arranged in terms of duration of therapy.

Since the presence of acute schizophrenic symptoms such as anxiety, hallucinations, delusion, fears, direct expression of conflicts, poor impulse control, depersonalization phenomena, and thought disorder is used as a criterion of initial diagnosis, these must also be assessed under one category. Two categories must be assigned to dynamic conflictive emotional/ attitudinal factors, interpersonal in one, self-evaluative in the other. These would include expansive-aggressive, self-effacing-dependent, and withdrawal attitudes, self-aggrandizing and self-denigrating evaluation. Since improvement is a function of the patient's involvement in therapy, factors indicating this must be evaluated as another category of variables. Here would be included such factors as self-interest and curiosity, initiative and spontaneity, psychic flexibility and mobility, awareness of and closeness to inner experiences and self-expressiveness. These attitudes would correspond roughly to what Rogers and his group[44] described as "process movement," changes in which were considered the essential index of positive outcome. Finally, since constructive growth is held to be the ultimate goal of therapy, one category of variables must include qualities like self-directedness (autonomy), ability to make choices, acceptance of consequences and responsibility, realistic self-image and identity, self-acceptance, productive and enjoyable activities as in work, sex, and interpersonal relationships, and a tolerance for the normal frustrations and conflict situations of life. As these categories have been arranged in our schema, changes in them would correspond grossly to the length of time in analytic therapy. Manifest symptoms might improve first, then greater involvement in therapy, attitudinal changes later, and so forth. Of course, this correlation is only a most approximate one, since the constant and fluctuating movement I have described in the "analytic process" is also occurring, and constructive growth is hopefully a basic aspect of all change during analysis, though it may occur more or less rapidly at different times.

In addition to being able to define and delineate such criteria, another implication is that they be measurable. This means, first, according to some "psychometrically respectable assessment instruments."[42] And, second, that the resulting statistical correlation between test figures and our behavioral-dynamic variables be expressible through some curvilinear relationship. The problem of finding suitable psychological procedures for measuring the specific variables relevant to our approach has proved most difficult and has been concerning us for the past year. We believe that we may have finally found a series of such scales, originally developed by other research groups, which can be modified for our purposes and easily administered. Such measures must respond to the question of initial severity of illness and degree of health, thereby establishing a base line for evaluation. It is only against such a standard that degree of change is assessable when measured at later intervals. Relative change is thus considered more relevant than absolute change. The uniqueness of the patient is thus respected rather than trying to fit him into a preconceived pigeonhole. Furthermore, the setting of such initial observable standards will depend, in final analysis, on the judgment and perceptiveness of the analyst; therefore, it will have to be compared with similar judgments by another independent, noninvolved screening analyst as well as by patient self-evaluative tests.

In conclusion, this concept of schizophrenia and its various implications offer many positive possibilities for the psychoanalytic treatment of these psychoses. We are hopeful that 5 yr. will provide some more definitive evidence of this, if our projected research program can be carried out as planned. The enormity of the problem and of the promise justifies the attempt.

References

1. Masserman, J.: Principles of Dynamic Psychiatry. Philadelphia, W. B. Saunders, 1946.
2. Schact, M., and Kempster, S.: Useful techniques in the treatment of patients with schizophrenia. Psychiatry 16:35, 1953.
3. Burnham, D., Gladstone, A., and Gidson, R.: Schizophrenia and the Need-Fear Dilemma. New York, International Universities Press, 1969.
4. Stierlin, H.: Conflict and Reconciliation: Human Relations and Schizophrenia. New York, Science House, 1969.
5. Rubins, J.: A holistic approach to the schizophrenias—Pt. I: Sociocultural, developmental and psychogenetic factors. Amer. J. Psychoanal. 25:131, 1969.
6. ———: A holistic approach to the schizophrenias—Pt. II: Psychodynamics of clinical symptoms. Amer. J. Psychoanal. 30:30, 1970.
7. ———: A holistic approach to the schizophrenias—Pt. III: The therapeutic process. Amer. J. Psychoanal. 32:16, 1972.
8. Mosher, L: Recent trends in the psychosocial treatment of schizophrenia. Amer. J. Psychoanal. 32:9, 1972.
9. Freud, S.: On narcissism. In: Collected Papers, Vol. IV. London, Hogarth, 1914.
10. Bychowski, G.: Psychotherapy of the Psychoses. New York, Grune & Stratton, 1952.
11. Federn, P.: Analysis of psychotics. Int. J. Psychoanal. 15:209, 1934.
12. Alexander, F.: Schizophrenic psychoses. Arch. Neurol. (Chicago) 26:815, 1931.
13. Schilder, P.: Scope of psychotherapy in schizophrenia. Amer. J. Psychiat. 11:1181, 1932.
14. Sechehaye, M.: Symbolic Realization. New York, International Universities Press, 1951.
15. Schwing, G.: A Way to the Soul of the Mentally Ill. New York, International Universities Press, 1954.
16. Azima, H.: Object-Relations Therapy of Schizophrenic States: Technique and Theory, Psychiatry Research Reports No. 17. Washington, D.C., American Psychiatric Association, 1963.
17. Rosen, J. N.: Direct Psychoanalytic Psychiatry. New York, Grune & Stratton, 1962.
18. Wechsler, M.: The structural problem in schizophrenia: Therapeutic implications. Int. J. Psychoanal. 32:157, 1951.
19. Boyer, L., and Giovacchini, P.: Psychoanalytic Treatment of Characterological and Schizophrenic Disorders. New York, Science House, 1967.
20. Spotnitz, H.: Modern Psychoanalysis of the Schizophrenic Patient. New York, Grune & Stratton, 1968.
21. Benedetti, G.: Analytische Psychotherapie der Psychoses. In: Hoff, H. (Ed.): Lehrbuch der Psychiatrie. Basel, Schwabe, 1956.

22. Muller, C.: Les therapeutiques analytiques des psychoses. Rev. Franc. Psychanal. 22:573, 1958.
23. Recamier, P. C.: Psychoanalytic therapy of the psychoses. In: Nacht, S. (Ed.): Psychoanalysis Today. New York, Grune & Stratton, 1959.
24. Sullivan, H. S.: Schizophrenia as a Human Process. New York, W. W. Norton, 1962.
25. Fromm-Reichmann, F.: Aspects of psychoanalytic psychotherapy with schizophrenics. In: Brody, E., and Redlich, F. (Eds.): Psychotherapy with Schizophrenics. New York, International Universities Press, 1952.
26. Powdermaker, F.: Concepts found useful in treatment of ambulatory schizophrenic patients. Psychiatry 15:61, 1952.
27. Searles, H.: Collected Papers on Schizophrenia. New York, International Universities Press, 1962.
28. Will, O.: Schizophrenia: Psychological treatment. In: Freedman, A., and Kaplan, H. (Eds.): Comprehensive Textbook of Psychiatry. Philadelphia, Williams & Wilkins, 1967.
29. Arieti, S.: Psychotherapy of schizophrenia. Arch. Gen. Psychiat. (Chicago) 6:20, 1962.
30. Kilpatrick, E.: On the treatment of schizophrenia (discussion). In: Rifkin, A. H. (Ed.): Schizophrenia in Psychoanalytic Office Practice. New York, Grune & Stratton, 1957.
31. Metzger, E.: On schizophrenia. Amer. J. Psychoanal. 17:114, 1957.
32. Hott, L.: On schizophrenia. Amer. J. Psychoanal. 17:118, 1957.
33. Boigon, M.: The psychoanalytic approach to the psychoses. Amer. J. Psychoanal. 26:72, 1966.
34. Sheiner, S.: On the therapy of schizophrenia. Amer. J. Psychoanal. 24:167, 1954; 25:158, 1965; 26:76, 1966.
35. Karon, B.: The resolution of acute schizophrenic reactions. A contribution to the development of non-classical psychotherapeutic techniques. Psychotherapy 1:27, 1963; 6:88, 1969.
36. May, P.: The Treatment of Schizophrenia. New York, Science House, 1968.
37. Rogers, C.: The Therapeutic Relationship and Its Impact: Psychotherapy with Schizophrenics. Madison, University of Wisconsin Press, 1957.
38. American Psychological Association: Research in Psychotherapy, Vol. I, Rubinstein, E., and Parloff, M. (Eds.): Vol. II, Strupp, H., and Luborsky, L. (Eds.); Vol. III, Schlien, J. (Ed.). Washington, D.C., American Psychological Association, 1958, 1961, 1966.
39. Shakow, D.: On doing research in schizophrenia. Arch. Gen. Psychiat. (Chicago) 20:618, 1969.
40. Committee on Research, Group for Advancement of Psychiatry: Psychiatric Research and the Assessment of Change. New York, Group for Advancement of Psychiatry, 1966.
41. Meltzoff, J., and Kornreich, M.: Research in Psychotherapy. New York, Grune & Stratton, 1970.
42. Strupp, H., and Bergin, A.: Some empirical and conceptual bases for coordinated research in psychotherapy. Int. J. Psychiat.
43. Whitehorn, J., and Betz, B.: Study of psychotherapeutic relationships between physicians and schizophrenic patients. Amer. J. Psychiat. 111:321, 1954; 117:215, 1960.

Discussion by Otto Allen Will, Jr., M.D.

In discussing prepsychotic maturational development Dr. Rubins refers to a variety of factors—organic defects, chemical or enzymatic dysfunctions, lowered anxiety tolerance, etc.—which may interfere with this process. It seems to me that such a remark might be made about all human development, which is fraught with many hazards and in which the appropriate sequential matching of ability with experience is so uncertain that many—perhaps most—human beings are but dim representations of what they might have become. The question of a possible organic defect related specifically to schizophrenia does not concern me here. Schizophrenia itself is so imprecisely defined that it is difficult to speak of etiology in terms of single events or conditions. I do not think that the so-called schizophrenia problems will be done away with through the discovery of some basic defect—as in the realms of chemistry and genetics; but, of course, I do not know what will come, and can only comment from an admittedly restricted point of view.

Schizophrenic behavior is—to me- -a form of human living and an expression of what has been, is, and can be anticipated in the life of the person concerned. I do not think that our primary task is to do away with this disorder—to eradicate it as some disease—for in so doing we might destroy an important and unique source of knowledge about ourselves. This is not to say that I somehow honor this state or look upon it as a superior or ennobling way of life. I do not. Schizophrenia is one of the miserable varieties of human compromise and enslavement; as we seek to be of help to the encaptured we must observe as best we can the processes in which they are involved, attempting thus to find an increase in freedom as we escape from the more dangerous of our self-created mythologies.

The author "postulates that schizophrenia is wholly defensive against the conflict of compulsive emotions or attitudes, both interpersonal and intrapsychic, in active dynamic opposition." He disagrees "with the concept of this psychosis as a 'collapse' of defenses with subsequent regression." The emphasis is on conflict.

In schizophrenic behavior each observer can find something of himself which suggests that such behavior is a distortion, intensification, or reduction of the commonplace, its very familiarity inviting a variety of responses—fascination, repulsion, avoidance, and often denial. It is not difficult in this field for each observer to find seeming confirmation for his theory—often abetted by patients who may discover that the production of "data" pleasing to the therapist (or others) may serve to reduce anxiety through keeping the peace. In a sense schizophrenia may be more simple than complex; by our concern with intricacy we may avoid the painful possibility that our look at "disease" is but a look at ourselves.

There follows a brief outline of a view of the development of schizophrenic behavior that emphasizes cultural-social-interpersonal influences and may not be significantly at variance with that which has been presented by Dr. Rubins.

1. In infancy—prior to the development of a defined concept of self, of dependable and clear object relations, and of speech skills—discomfort (ill defined and the forerunner of anxiety) is experienced, disturbing the beginning sense of trust and confidence in self and others, and requiring the use of functions such as denial, dissociation, and alterations of the body image and self-concept.

2. Behavior acquired later—including such symbol operations as speech—may be put to use as "defenses," usually interfering with communication and learning as it serves to reduce anxiety.

3. Although learning defects acquired in one era of growth interfere with progress in subsequent eras, corrective experience can alter the course of events favorably. My guess is that many a person does not reach the schizophrenic condition because of fortunate interpersonal contacts during, or prior to, adolescence.

4. In adolescence skills must be refined and tasks performed that require a fuller expression of the personality than previously demanded. I refer to such matters as the forming of intimate and freely communicative relationships, the patterning of sexual behavior, separation from the family, selection of career, acceptance of a dependable self-identity, and so on.

5. The young person must again deal with two basic human problems—attachment and separation. He must leave or modify some alliances with people and ideas and be able to form and accept others. The integration of an intimate relationship requires revelation—of the self to others and to the self of aspects of experience hitherto dissociated or denied. The entrance into awareness of sentiments long dormant is an awakening into nightmare—a state of panic in which the boundaries of self and thought are for the time being beyond control.

6. The person so described must act with urgency to solve an undefined problem. Perhaps the problem is something like this: human relatedness is a necessity for survival and is also the apparent source of destruction. How does one maintain the required minimum of meaningful communication, keep in contact with others, hold anxiety to a tolerable level, and avoid being publicly identified as mad and thus even more unsuitable and undesirable?

7. From the point of view presented here schizophrenic behavior may be looked upon as problem oriented, purposive, and goal directed. In this sense schizophrenia is not only madness—but method—which is not to say that all of its performances are to be interpreted, fully understood, or decoded. Some of the speech of the schizophrenic person, for example, may (like that of any of us) be decorative and playful rather than informative.

Therapy

In the section on treatment Dr. Rubins refers to the use of drugs as an adjunct to psychotherapy. I am chary in the use of such agents, but this is a subject by itself. At times drugs may be use- for sleep, but when possible I prefer that the human relationship be substituted for the chemical when the goal is to limit anxiety and facilitate communication. I refer here to the acutely disturbed adolescent or young adult patient cared for in a residential setting by a competent staff whose efforts are well coordinated. Such work is for a group—not for the therapist alone. What I wish to avoid is the dulling of perception and the nuances of emotion and the possible interference with learning that may occur when drugs are used to control behavior.

A patient may be given drugs less to allay his own suffering than to reduce that of the staff. Such action can be acceptable if its motivation is clearly recognized. Better yet, however, attention should be turned to strengthening of the staff through education, personal therapy, and relief from excessive pressure of work.

The milieu is at one point spoken of as ancillary to individual psychotherapy. I think that the milieu is a major factor in the therapeutic process. In the institution the patient may have the opportunity to expand his social skills through participation with peers and others in groups of different sizes, and if he lives in his own family or not, some form of therapeutic contact with the family can be advantageous.

Dr. Rubins' discussion of the therapist's role is a helpful contribution to a difficult subject. That role is unique and not easy to describe; it contains attributes of other roles, but it is none of these—it is itself. There are certain major characteristics of the psychotherapeutic task:

1. An attachment must be formed in which a wide range of sentiments can be expressed and an enduring sense of trust developed.

2. The therapist must be able to endure discovering how other people view life and how they came to form such views—perhaps at great and painful variance with those of the therapist.

3. As the patient's goals and values are identified and clarified he is helped to accept their attainment, modification, or abandonment in accordance with his abilities and opportunities.

4. The process has a quality of mutuality but the relationship is not that of friends —it is more.

5. As attachment is a fundamental aspect of the task, so is separation. One cannot exist without the other.

A parent, a teacher, and a psychotherapist have—if they are to continue in the work with sufficient satisfaction—certain qualities in common. They can form an attachment, can foster dependency without exploiting it, can derive pleasure from the growth of another, and can accept departure and change as essential attributes of life —and love.

Research

In speaking of research in psychotherapy, perhaps the simplest thing to say is that it is a difficult task that often appears to be incomprehensible or impossible. I am of the opinion that resarch is not required to demonstrate that the human relationship is of vital importance to human beings—schizophrenic or otherwise. Psychotherapy is a form of relationship designed to permit and facilitate a wide range of behavioral expression and observation without lasting hurt to the participants, thus advancing learning and the ability to seek, select, and make use of available experience. Research can be designed to study the form of the relationship, its course, and ways in which it can be destructive as well as otherwise.

The research design devised by Dr. Rubins and his associates requires a more sophisticated comment than I am able to give. The proposal is to compare by certain criteria the progress of several patient groups, each subjected to a particular form of therapy: (a) psychoanalysis; (b) drugs; (c) milieu (day care); (d) a combination of the above; and (e) "no therapy."

I think that there will be many overlapping factors in these groups and I should not be willing to use this study as somehow a test of the human relationship as it functions in psychotherapy and schizophrenia.

I continue to favor further use of the single case as a method of study. I know that such accounts can be anecdotal and unreliable, but carefully kept records can reveal the development of patterns of behavior and the possible relationship of these to the operations of the therapist, other staff personnel, family members, influences of the past, and so on. The therapist's additions of information as to his own experience from day to day can be illuminating—and not put aside as a form of counter-analysis. If the relationship is interpersonal—which it is—the therapist cannot be omitted from its study, despite the possible discomfort of embarrassment and the evolving of a truly humble stance.

In conclusion, I consider the psychotherapeutic task with schizophrenic patients to be—potentially, at least—well worth the expenditure of energy, time, money, and personal distress. A few people can be helped with what we do—but I think these few can help all of us a great deal. The schizophrenic person presents to us with startling clarity aspects of human living often otherwise concealed or ignored. I refer to problems of attachment, dependency, dissociation, body imagery, aggression, fear, anxiety, the use of symbols, grief, denial, separation, and so on. The contributions that can be made through our efforts to the general human good may be small— and yet significant. We need not despise what we are able to do professionally because it is limited and because in the rush of man toward an unknown destiny our efforts may be unnoted or put aside. In our work we are not required to be optimistic or pessimistic—only observant and courageous enough to report—and perhaps act upon—what we see, or think we see.

part 4

CLINICAL STUDIES

An Evaluation of Interviewer Bias*

CARL I. WOLD, PH. D.

NORMAN TABACHNICK, M.D.

The problem of bias

This paper is a report of an investigation of interviewer bias during a psychoanalytic study of suicide and self-destructiveness in automobile accidents.

What is meant by interviewer bias, and why are we concerned with it in this research? The issue arises when we consider the task of the interviewer. He explores the hypotheses of our study during psychoanalytic interviews with the subjects. From this experience, the interviewer is asked to gather data and make judgments about the subjects which he reports on a structured data sheet. Bias is here regarded as attitudes or preconceptualizations or hypotheses of the interviewer which relate to the phenomena under study. These biases, if present, may or may not influence the findings of the study.

Matarazzo[1] reviewed studies of interviewer bias. Earlier studies were

* This research is a portion of a larger study of suicide and accidents, under the direction of Norman Tabachnick, M.D., supported by National Institute of Mental Health Grant DH 15510.

reported in the area of social science research. Hollingworth[2] and others demonstrated interviewer bias in employment situations. Rice[3] reported interviewer bias among 12 trained social workers in their interviews with applicants for social welfare. It was found that the interviewers' feelings about ill effects of drinking and feelings about the social system influenced their responses to a group of drinkers. The age and sex of interviewers has been reported as a source of bias by Hyman.[4]

More relevant to this accident research are the findings of Raines and Rohrer.[5, 6] They studied the role of interviewer bias in psychiatric interviews. In the first study, using 9 experienced Navy psychiatrists, they reached two conclusions: (1) that two psychiatrists, each interviewing the same man, observed different personality traits in this man and also reported different dominant defense mechanisms used by him in his everyday behavior, and (2) that any given psychiatrist had a preferred personality type classification which he utilized more frequently than on a chance basis, with different psychiatrists preferring different personality-type categories. When 5 of the psychiatrists reinterviewed the subjects 5 wk. later (no psychiatrist interviewing the man he had previously seen), the same biases obtained.

The authors concluded that a clinical interviewer's subject served as a projective device for the interviewer and reflected significant aspects of the psychiatrist's own personality. They felt that each psychiatrist's own life experiences made him more sensitive to certain facets of the patient's dynamics and made him perceptually distort other facets of the patient.

In their second study, Raines and Rohrer had other psychiatrists make independent assessments of the interviewer. They demonstrated a correlation between independently judged facets of the personality of the interviewer and the interviewer's reports of his subjects.

In our study, bias might play a role during the psychoanalytic interviewing of the subjects. Bias might be influential not only during the interview or data gathering but in the way the data were reported as well. Primarily, a structured data sheet was used by the interviewer to make public the findings of the interview. Bias was both controlled for and measured during this study, as reported below.

Controlling interviewer bias

It is likely that the psychoanalytic training of the interviewers provided one control of bias in this study. A fundamental tenet of the psychoanalytic method is that the analyst's awareness of his own conscious and unconscious biases allow him to make patient-centered observations. In spite of this control, however, the interviewer's bias might significantly influence the findings of this study.

Further control over bias was provided by the design and development of the data sheet. Most of the items required structured, objective answers in an attempt to minimize or eliminate ambiguous responses and highly interpretive data. Research with projective techniques [7, 8] has amply illustrated that individual bias is more evident in responses to unstructured stimuli.

The interrater reliability of the items in the data sheet provides another control of bias. All research interviews were voice recorded, and each interviewer's data sheet answers were compared with independent ratings of the recorded interviews. On this basis, as the study developed, items were changed or eliminated with the goal of using only the highly reliable items.

For each of the 205 items on the data sheet, the percent agreement between the answer given by the interviewer and those of independent raters was calculated. Table 1 shows the average (mean) percent agreement between interviews and independent raters, over all items, at the conclusion of the data gathering.

Table 1. Average (Mean) Percent Agreement

Actual *accident* cases ($n = 24$)	77%
Actual *suicide* cases ($n = 29$)	76%
Actual *appendectomy* cases ($n = 31$)	78%
Overall cases ($n = 84$)	77%

Analysis of variance of the interviewer-rater percent agreement showed that any differences were not statistically significant. What this means is that the answers given by interviewers filling out the data sheet were very much in agreement with answers of the raters who listened to the interviews on tape and completed the data sheet independently. At this juncture, we had no reason to feel that interviewer bias had influenced the findings of the study.

Measuring interviewer bias

In addition to controlling bias, we utilized the following procedure to measure bias as well. All psychoanalytic interviewers and independent raters were asked to complete a data sheet for a hypothetical subject from each of the experimental categories. These data sheets for hypothetical subjects were obtained before the actual experimental interviews with real subjects and again upon completion of the interviewing phase of the research.

Instructions to interviewers for the hypothetical "accident person" were: Fill out a data sheet to represent a typical one-car driver automobile accident victim. He should be between the ages of 18 and 45 yr., male, and have been seriously injured in the accident. There are no other restrictions on your formulations.

Instructions for the hypothetical "suicide person" were : Fill out a data sheet to represent a typical suicide attempt victim. He should be between the ages of 18 and 45 yr., male, and have made a near-lethal suicide attempt. There are no other restrictions on your formulations.

Instructions for the hypothetical "appendectomy person" were: Fill out a data sheet to represent a typical appendectomy patient. He should be between the ages of 18 and 45 yr., male, and have just undergone an operation which was a confirmed appendectomy. There are no other restrictions on your formulations.

To what extent did the interviewers begin the study with a shared conceptual bias about the subjects whom they were to interview? Table 2 shows the average (mean) percent agreement among all psychoanalytic interviewers for their initial description of hypothetical accident, suicide, and appendectomy subjects.

Table 2. Average (Mean) Percent Agreement (Before Interviewing Actual Subjects)

Hypothetical accident cases ($n = 16$)	60%
Hypothetical suicide cases ($n = 16$)	62%
Hypothetical appendectomy cases ($n = 16$)	75%

There was a good deal of agreement among the interviewers' descriptions of hypothetical subjects. In large measure, interviewers began the project with shared conceptual biases about a prototypic accident subject, suicide subject, and appendectomy subject.

Was there a correspondence between the interviewers' preconceptualizations and what they actually found during the research interviews? Table 3 shows rank order correlations (Rhos) between the percent agreement among interviewers on hypothetical cases with their agreement on the actual cases.

Table 3. Rank Order Correlation (Rho)

Hypothetical vs. actual accident cases	0.08 (not significant)
Hypothetical vs. actual suicide cases	0.13 (not significant)
Hypothetical vs. actual appendectomy cases	0.11 (not significant)

These correlations were all statistically nonsignificant, indicating that there was very little agreement between the interviewers' initial bias and the descriptions of actual subjects. Apparently the initial bias had not been imposed upon the actual data.

In order to assess in more detail the correspondence between the interviewers' answers about hypothetical subjects and the data from actual subjects, comparisons were made item by item for the entire data sheet. Table 4 shows the number of items which interviewers judged to discriminate between accident, suicide, and appendectomy subjects.

Table 4. Number of Items Judged to Discriminate Between Accident, Suicide, and Appendectomy Subjects

Hypothetical subjects (before interviewing actual subjects)	126
Actual subjects	50
Characteristic of both hypothetical and actual subjects	27

It can be seen that the interviewers judged a large number of items differentially among hypothetical accident, suicide, and appendectomy subjects. In fact, among actual subjects during the research, only 40 items differentiated among the three experimental groups. Only 27 items, which were judged significant among hypothetical subjects, turned out to be significant among the actual subjects. This finding further substantiates the discrepancy between the interviewers' initial bias and the empirical findings with actual subjects. An inspection of the items themselves reveals that hypothetical accident subjects were described by the interviewers as similar to hypothetical suicide subjects and quite different from hypothetical appendectomy subjects. This is in contradistinction to the main findings of the research. Ratings of the actual subjects showed similarity between the accident and appendectomy subjects; both groups were different from the suicide group.

Had the interviewers' initial bias been influenced by the actual interviewing experience? As noted above, interviewers completed data sheets for hypothetical subjects once again upon completion of their interviews with actual subjects. When these data sheets were compared with the original hypothetical ratings completed before the actual interviewing was initiated, no statistically significant changes had occurred (using an analysis-of-variance test). In spite of their experience with actual subjects which produced findings to challenge their initial biases, interviewers maintained their initial biases substantially unchanged.

Discussion

It was not surprising that the psychoanalytic interviewers entered the experimental situation with shared conceptual biases about subjects whom they were to interview. In addition to having rather homogeneous professional background and training, all the psychoanalytic interviewers were members of the same training institute and part of an ongoing research seminar interested in automobile accident in the context of developing a more general psychoanalytic theory of action. Initial agreement about hypothetical appendectomy cases was even closer than the agreement among hypothetical accident and hypothetical suicide cases. On examination of the individual item, it seemed that the reason for the consistency among interviewers (their initial bias) toward appendectomy cases was the fact that most of the items on the data sheet were in a pathologic direction, and most of the interviewers gave "no" answers for hypothetical appendectomy cases. This meant that the interviewers came to this study with the belief that appendectomy subjects would show little psychopathology, which resulted in consistent answers among interviewers on the data sheet.

Interviewers had the initial bias that the actual accident subjects would be more similar to the actual suicide subjects than to the appendectomy subjects. They believed that strong, self-destructive personality factors characterized accident victims, were important in the etiology of the accident, and were analogues of components of the suicidal state. There had been prior research evidence to support these biases.[9-11] In fact, during actual research interviewing, the interviewers were confronted with subjects who gave little evidence to support the initial biases. This was reported by the interviewers on the data sheet, although contrary to their biases.

How did the interviewers conceptualize the discrepancy between the empirical data of this study and their initial biases? When bias was measured once again upon completion of the research, it had changed little from the initial position. This finding was supported during debriefing meetings with all interviewers. Most interviewers felt that self-destructive components are to be found among accident subjects in spite of the negative indications of this research. They felt that the data sheet itself had inhibited the finding of self-destructive trends among accident subjects by failing to capture and make public the deeper and more important dimensions of their psychoanalytic interviews.

In conclusion, some speculations can be made about the importance of the findings:

1. Psychoanalysts are able to identify and report data about research subjects independent of their expectations, even contrary to their bias.

2. Psychoanalysts maintain certain biases in spite of contrary empirical data.

3. Rigorous, empirical methods are necessary and important adjuncts to psychoanalytic research.

4. There is no reason not to believe that thes findings apply to other social scientists and interviewers as well.

References

1. Matarazzo, J. B.: The Interview. In: Wolman, B. B. (Ed.): The Handbook of Clinical Psychology. New York, McGraw-Hill, 1965.
2. Hollingworth, H. L.: Judging Human Character. New York, Appleton and Croft, 1922.
3. Rice, S.: Contagious bias in the interview: A methodological note, Amer. J. Sociol. 35:420–423, 1929.
4. Hyman, H. H.: Interviewing in Social Research. Chicago, University of Chicago Press, 1954.
5. Raines, J. N., and Rohrer, J. H.: The operational matrix of psychiatric practice: Consistency and variability in interview impressions in different psychiatrists. Amer. J. Psychiat. 111:721–733, 1965.
6. Raines, J. N., and Rohrer, J. H.: The operational matrix of psychiatric practice: Variability in psychiatric impressions and the projection hypothesis. Amer. J. Psychiat. 117:133–139, 1960.
7. Bell, J. E.: Projective Techniques. New York, Longmans, Green and Company, 1948.
8. Ainsworth, M. D.: Problems of validation. In Klopfer, B., Ainsworth, M. D., Klopfer, W. G., and Holt, R. R. (Eds.): Developments in the Rorschach Technique, Vol. I. New York World Book Co., 1954.
9. Tabachnick, N.: The psychology of fatal accidents. In: Shneidman, E. (Ed.): Essays in Self-destruction. New York, Science House, 1967.
10. Litman, R. E., and Tabachnick, N.: Fatal one-car accidents. Psychoanal. Quart. 36:248–259, 1967.
11. Tabachnick, N., Litman, R. E., Osman, M., Jones, W. L., Cohn, J., Kasper, A., and Moffat, J.: Comparative psychiatric study of accidental and suicidal death. Arch. Gen. Psychiat. (Chicago) 14:60–68, 1966.

The Telepathic Dream: Experimental Findings and Clinical Implications

MONTAGUE ULLMAN, M.D.

If psi (paranormal) events occur it is reasonable to assume that they serve or did serve some time in the distant past a significant function for the organism involved. Evidence has been gathered from analytic practice in support of the existence of such events, particularly in the form of the telepathic dream. The study of these dreams in a psychodynamic context has also yielded a number of interesting speculative hypotheses as to their meaning and the circumstances of their occurrence.[1,2] What this amounts to in terms of my own experience is that, if not all patients, at least some, can, when necessary, mobilize something analogous to an unconscious paranormal radar system capable of alerting them to impending interpersonal danger. This generally

The studies reported were supported by the following foundations: The Mary Reynolds Babcock Foundation, The Foundation for the Study of Consciousness, The Irving F. Laucks Foundation, The New Horizons Foundation, The Society for Comparative Philosophy, and The W. Clement and Jessie V. Stone Foundation.

The author wishes to express his appreciation to Dr. Stanley Krippner, director of the Dream Laboratory at the Maimonides Medical Center, for his help in the preparation of this paper based on the work of the Laboratory.

comes about when countertransferential feelings rise to the surface or other factors interfere with the rapport between therapist and patient.

Partisans of a regressive theory of psi events view such happenings as isolated breakthroughs of an archaic communication system at times of stress or decompensation.[3] At the other extreme are those who favor the view that psi factors enter into all communicative processes but that in the ordinary course of events they are not attended to.[4] Regardless of which theory proves to be correct, the fact remains that when the individual by virtue of limiting psychological or emotional factors fails to maintain his sense of effective participation in the here-and-now psi effects become more visible. The more fragile and vulnerable one's hold on reality, the more often and more striking were the paranormal occurrences.

The above speculations seemed to be borne out by clinical observations made by myself and others. In 1949[5] I wrote: ". . . Very ill individuals teetering on the brink but not yet over on the psychotic side often indicate remarkable Psi ability in the course of analysis," but ". . . once psychosis, or the complete absence of effective relationships with other people, sets in the indications at present are that at least in the experimental situation Psi functioning is not remarkable, nor is it in the clinical situation in my own experience. . . ." Finally I called attention to ". . . the consistent clinical fact that psychotics in their fantasies make elaborate pretensions at Psi ability, sometimes quite openly, sometimes in a more disguised form." In the light of this formulation psi functioning comes into being as a last desperate level of relatedness when personality factors interfere with more effective contact. Once the individual has withdrawn from the struggle to maintain his sense of relatedness, fantasy takes over and there are delusions of telepathy rather than any genuine demonstrable paranormal ability.

Quite recently I received a letter from someone unknown to me in which the following passage occurred:

> One aspect of ESP which intrigues me is its apparent enhancement in acutely psychotic individuals. A writer friend and I, both of whom had once had schizophrenic episodes, had discussed at length the paranormal perception that seemed to rear its improbable head from time to time during the psychosis.
>   Your remark about this phenomenon in the *Psychic* interview was the first commentary I had seen in print.
>   I've also noticed that the physiological phenomena of meditation—especially the "electrified" feeling one sometimes gets—resemble the early euphoric stages of acute schizophrenia. Schizophrenics in the casebooks seem to have the illusion, at any rate, that they are "getting messages," and frequently think they're being bombarded by some sort of outside electricity.
>   Would it not be possible that the phenomena sometimes *contribute* to the

disordered thinking, adding to the confusion, rather than necessarily deriving from it?

The above is the first explicit acknowledgement to come to my attention, from someone who had experienced a schizophrenic episode, having a bearing on the possible accuracy of the speculative hypothesis offered above concerning the interrelation of psi events and psychotic process.

The evidence from the consulting room, as might be expected, was inadequate to the very difficult task of shifting the interest in psi events into the mainstream of science. More than personal testimony and evidential accounts were needed to take seriously a set of phenomena which on the face of it seemed so difficult to explain in terms of currently accepted models of the physical universe. It was with this in mind that I joined ranks with other parapsychologists similarly concerned with the problem of scientific credibility and undertook an experimental approach that began in the pre-REM era but which had to await the availability of the REM technology before it could be applied practically and systematically.[6] In this presentation I will briefly summarize the work of our laboratory and discuss some of the implications for psychoanalysis.

Methodology

The details of the procedures have been given in numerous earlier publications. In brief, for the sleep-telepathy experiments, which are the only ones summarized here, we worked either with single subjects over a period of 7 or 8 nights or with a series of subjects each sleeping in the laboratory for 1 night. Subjects were volunteers, some of whom were selected on the basis of earlier successful performances on screening nights. The subject's sleep was monitored and he was awakened at the estimated end of each REM period to report his dream. An agent or sender spent the night in a separate room attempting to telepathically influence the subject's dreams by concentrating on the selected target picture at intervals throughout the night and particularly when signaled that an REM period for the subject had begun. The target, generally an art print, was randomly selected by the agent from a pool of targets in opaque, sealed containers after the subject was in bed. Only the agent was aware of the target chosen for the particular night, and he remained in his room throughout the night acoustically isolated from both subject and experimenter. The dream protocols were transcribed from the taped reports. Copies of them, along with copies of the targets used for any given experimental series, were given to three or four independent judges who assessed correspondences on a blind basis. The results were analyzed using either the Latin-square analysis of variance technique or the application of the binomial expansion theorem.

Summaries of seven completed experiments are given. Four of these yielded statistically significant findings.

1. The first screening study. For this study, 12 volunteer subjects (*Ss*) spent 1 night each at the laboratory. Two staff members, 1 male and 1 female, alternated as Agents (*As*), attempting to influence *Ss'* dreams by means of telepathy. Target materials were famous art prints, randomly selected for each night once *Ss* had gone to bed. On the following morning, *Ss* were asked to match their dream recall against the entire collection of target pictures, selecting the art print which most closely corresponded to their dreams and ranking the other in descending order of correspondence. Four outside Judges (*Js*) followed a similar procedure; statistically significant data emerged from *Ss'* rankings and from one of the *J* evaluations. Significant differences between *As* were also obtained, with the 6 *Ss* paired with the male *A* obtaining closer target-dream correspondences than the 6 *Ss* working with the female *A*.[7]

2. The first Erwin study. Dr. W. Erwin, the *S* whose target-dream correspondences were the most direct in the first study, was paired with the male *A* from the screening study for a 7-night series. Statistically significant results were obtained from both *S*'s evaluation and the means of similar evaluations done by 3 *Js*.[8]

3. The second screening study. Twelve different *Ss* and two *As* were utilized in another 12-night series. The results did not attain statistical significance for either *S* or *Js*.[9]

4. The Posin study. Dr. R. Posin, who participated in the above study, was paired with the *A* she had worked with during her night in the laboratory. Neither *S* nor *Js* produced significant data for this 8-night series.[10]

5. The Grayeb study. T. Grayeb, another *S* from the same study, was selected for this 16-night study. Without the knowledge of *S*, *A* concentrated on a target during 8 nights of the study; for the other 8 nights these was neither an agent nor a target. The condition was determined randomly once *S* had gone to bed. Neither condition produced significant results.[11]

6. The second Erwin study. Dr. W. Erwin was again paired with the *A* from the second study for an 8-night series. The art print was accompanied by a box of "multisensory" materials on each night to enhance the emotionality of the target. For example, Daumier's painting "Advice to a Young Artist" was accompanied by a canvas and paints to enable *A* to "act out" the artist's role. No *S* evaluation was accomplished for this study. Analysis of the means of the 3 *Js'* evaluations produced significant results.[12]

7. *The Van de Castle study.* Dr. R. Van de Castle, a *S* who had produced several direct target-dream correspondences in a telepathy study at another laboratory,[13] was allowed to select his own *A* from the laboratory staff during the 8-night series. He selected a total of 3 *A*s: 1 for a single night, 1 for 2 nights, and 1 for 5 nights. Both *S*'s evaluations and those of an outside *J* were statistically significant.[14]

The following examples illustrate some of the correspondences noted between target and dreams. Excerpts from the dream reports and postsleep interviews are presented, with especially striking transcript-target correspondence italicized. It should be remembered that the judges worked from the entire dream transcript, not just the excerpts presented here.

Example 1

Target. "The Dark Figure," a painting by Castellon (Fig. 1). This painting portrays four people, one of them garbed in a somber, dark-brown gown. There are four round hoops above the figures; the hoops are held in the air by distorted children's hands. In the background is a red brick wall.

First dream report. "... For some reason I've been thinking of *a*

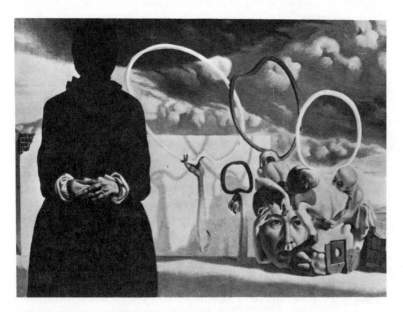

Fig. 1. "The Dark Figure," courtesy of the Whitney Museum of American Art.

barrel, . . . you know, *spinning around.* . . . There was some kind of activity or motion going on. *The barrel was spinning* . . . *like spinning in a circle.* . . . *It was like spinning. A top. Clockwise, left to right.* . . . *Dark-brown* wooden color. . . . *A red wheel spinning around.*"

Second dream report. " . . . I thought I saw lights and these lights were arranged in almost a *circular fashion.* . . . *You have a circle again* and there was some movement there. . . ."

Sixth dream report. " . . . There was a photograph I was looking at and in this photograph there was a bunch of people standing, and out front *there were four people in costumes* whose picture we were taking. . . . They were just posing . . . and looked pretty ridiculous. . . ."

Postsleep interview. " . . . . All I remember at first, I think, was these wooden *barrels, maybe three or four.* . . . *There was the iron rim going around the middle* to hold the slats together, and . . . *going around and around, spinning like a top.* . . . I also remember something about pale greenish-white lights. . . . *They formed kind of like an arch as though they started to spiral or circle* . . . *swirling like whirlpools.* . . . This photograph was rather a big one and it had *these young guys in costumes.* . . . Two summers ago *when I went to that camp for retarded children, they asked me to put on skits and costumes.* . . . *There are a lot of circling and spiraling effects in my dreams,* so any combination of effects like those I would look for in the target."

Example 2

Target. "The Seven Spinal Chakras," a painting by M. K. Scrailian (Fig. 2). This painting portrays a yogi involved in meditation while in the "lotus position." The seven chakras are portrayed on his spinal column and a beam of energy is directed upward from his head.

Third dream report. "I was very interested in research, natural communication—that is, using *natural energy* to serve it. . . . *I was talking to this guy who said he'd invented a way of using solar energy* and he showed me this box which was, I guess, about 3 ft. long and a foot square and it was perforated metal . . . and it had a handle on the top and inside there was a reflector screen to catch *the light from the sun which was all we needed to generate and store the energy,* and I think in some ways to amplify it and in which it was converted to battery source—something of that kind. . . . Anyway, it's pretty far out."

Postsleep interview summary. "I'm remembering a dream I had, I think in the first dream series I had in 1969, in which I had dreamed about *an energy box,* and the target picture turned out to be *a spinal column* which is sort of transmutation, because it turned out I had something wrong with

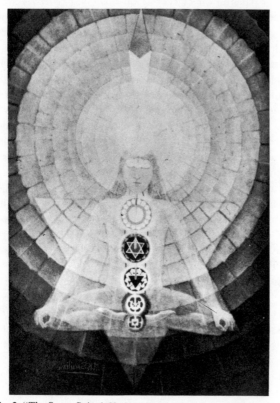

Fig. 2. "The Seven Spinal Chakras," courtesy of the Philosophical Research Society.

my own back and it was discovered by somebody who was a chiropractor, who just used manipulation to . . . correct it. I don't know whether this previous experience has any bearing on this at all."

Discussion

The results of these experiments have been discussed elsewhere from a parapsychological point of view. They raise a number of questions that should be of interest for psychoanalytic theory and practice.

First and foremost, perhaps, is the question raised earlier concerning the possible relation of psi events to psychopathological processes. Working with healthy subjects as we did and relying on a quantitative assessment of the data rather than on an analytic and interpretive approach, we got results that have no direct bearing on this question. They are, however, relevant indirectly insofar as they lend support to the psi hypothesis. In the one study (No. 7) where the dream material was explored in depth, targets dealing with the themes of aggression and sex had a greater telepathic impact. This would be in line with the evidence from both anecdotal and clinical sources that psi events are linked to affective processes. One could further speculate as to their linkage to problems of survival both for the individual and for the race.

At a practical level there are clear-cut technical and instrumental gains when there is explicit recognition of the psi hypothesis and its possible application in the therapeutic situation. Eisenbud is the foremost exponent of this point of view. As he notes, anyone sensitive to the occurrence of such psi effects would be in a position to recognize and handle countertransferential difficulties more promptly and more honestly. The work of Jourard[15] shows that self-disclosure is a powerful factor in accounting for the level of disclosure offered by others. Psi events make it possible to engage in a deeper level of mutual disclosure when such disclosure is relevant to the therapeutic situation.

There is one perhaps somewhat tangential but nevertheless relevant aspect to the work on telepathy. Those of us who have taken a public position espousing the reality of psi events are aware of a lost batallion of people who are in distress and wish to seek psychiatric help but who hold back out of fear of rebuff. They are people who have had psi experiences they consider to be both genuine and either central to their problem or related to it. They fear exposing themselves to an entrenched bias while at the same time recognizing their need for an objective assessment and help. Many of them know from the kind of past experience they have had along the straight psychiatric route that no credence is to be expected and that what they have experienced as valid is received as if it could not be anything but pathological. Caught in this kind of bind, many such individuals ultimately gravitate toward fringe groups in search of the support they need.

Conclusion

The work of our laboratory represents the first systematic experimental investigation of the telepathic dream. The data developed thus far do support the telepathy hypotheses. Of the attempts to replicate the Maimonides experiments, one has been successful,[16] two have been unsuccessful,[17,18] and one has produced an equivocal result.[19] All four studies represented the investigators' initial attempts to study this phenomenon, and it is difficult to conjecture what the results would have been if a long-range study had been planned.

References

1. Devereux, G. (Ed.): Psychoanalysis and the Occult. New York, International Universities Press, 1943.
2. Eisenbud, J.: Psi and Psychoanalysis. New York, Grune & Stratton, 1970.
3. Price, H. H.: Psychical research and human personality. Hibbert J. 47:105–113, 1949.
4. Thouless, R. H., and Wiesner, B. P.: The psi processes in normal and paranormal psychology. J.Parapsychol. 12:192–212, 1948.
5. Ullman, M.: On the nature of psi processes. J. Parapsychol. 13:1, 1949.
6. Ullman, M., and Krippner, S.: Dream Studies and Telepathy: An Experimental Approach. Parapsychological Monographs No 12. New York, Parapsychology Foundation, 1970.
7. Ullman, M., Krippner, S., and Feldstein, S.: Experimentally-induced telepathic dreams: Two studies using EEG-REM monitoring techniques. Int. J. Parapsychol. 8:577–603, 1966.
8. Ullman, M., Krippner, S., and Feldstein, S.: Experimentally-induced telepathic dreams: Two studies using EEG-REM monitoring technique. Int. J. Neuropsychiat. 2:420–437, 1966.
9. Ullman, M.: Telepathy and dreams. Exp. Med. Surg. 27:19–38, 1969.
10. Ullman, M., and Krippner, S.: *Op. cit.*
11. *Ibid.*
12. Ullman, M., and Krippner, S.: A laboratory approach to the nocturnal dimension of paranormal experience: Report of a confirmatory study using the REM monitoring technique. Biol. Psychiat. 1:259–270, 1969.
13. Hall, C.: Experimente zur Telepathischen Beeinflussung von Traumen. Parapsychol. Grenzgebiete Psychol. 10:18–47, 1967.
14. Krippner, S., and Ullman, M.: Telepathy and dreams: A controlled experiment with electroencephalogram-electro-oculogram monitoring. J. Nerv. Ment. Dis. 151:394–403, 1970.
15. Jourard, S. M.: Self-Disclosure, An Experimental Analysis of the Transparent Self. New York, John Wiley & Sons, 1971.
16. Hall, C.: Experimente zur Telepathischen Beeinflussung von Träumen. Parapsychol. Grenzgebiete Psychol. 10: 18–47, 1967.
17. Belvedere, E., and Foulkes, D.: Telepathy and dreams: A failure to replicate. Percept. Motor Skills 33:783–789, 1971.
18. Strauch, I.: Zur Methodik Telepathischer Traumexperimente. Parapsychol. Grenzgebiete Psychol. 8:55, 1965.
19. Globus, G. G., Knapp, P. H., Skinner, J. C., and Healy, G.: An appraisal of telepathic communication in dreams (abstract). Psychophysiology 4:365, 1968.

Psychosocial Aspects of Medical Practice: Primary Physicians in a Changing Urban Neighborhood*

MAURICE R. GREEN, M.D.
ESTHER HAAR, M.D.
LYON HYAMS, M.S., M.D.

Introduction

Because we are concerned with the changing role of the primary physician in relation to his patients and to psychiatry, we have attempted to clarify the role conflicts and conflicting expectations physicians experience with their patients and with psychiatrists. We will describe the results of a large study dealing with the way doctors view their roles and with their ideal expectations of themselves and of psychiatrists and then describe in more detail a smaller study of doctors in a rapidly changing urban area so as to illustrate the issues presented.

With the increasing urbanization of America, its rapid technological development, and its great population increase, the nature of the relationship of medicine to society is questioned more and more in professional and lay circles. It has become increasingly evident that physicians as well

*Supported by U.S. Public Health Service Research Grant IR01 MH 16624-01 from the National Institutes of Health, Bethesda, Md., at the William Alanson White Institute, New York.

147

as patients work in an historical and social context that shapes the form and appearance of disease as well as the nature of its treatment. This is especially true of psychiatric and emotional illness—so much so that some psychiatrists question the appropriateness of the term illness itself and suggest euphemisms such as "games people play" or "problems in living."

The primary physician in a contemporary city must cope not only with the crises of urban change and deterioration that challenge every major city today, but also with the effects these changes have on his relationship to his patients. He is confronted with these matters directly in his everyday practice of medicine, whether they are overtly presented to him as complaints of a psychiatric nature or covertly presented as somatic symptoms indicative of stressful life circumstances and painful emotional relationships.[1] He is called upon by the government, by his medical associations, and by psychiatric groups to attempt a comprehensive medical approach that includes attention to social problems of violence, drugs, and alcoholism, cooperation with community mental health centers and aftercare programs, and management of the psychiatric aspects of medical and surgical procedures.

Role models of medical care

This paper will address itself first to the conflicting expectations regarding the role of primary physicians, including specialists, family physicians, and general practitioners in their relation to their patients and to their psychiatric colleagues. We define the primary physician as the physician first consulted by the patient, and who, therefore, has the responsibility for the overall treatment plan or referral, where indicated.

Over the centuries, in our culture, three broad models have characterized the relationship between the physician and his patient: the wise, magical healer, such as the shaman; the skilled, detached scientist, such as the radiologist or surgeon; and the expert partner, such as a ski instructor or a psychoanalyst.

Physicians have traditionally worn a mantle of moral authority interwoven with strong threads of ritual and custom. This role was derived from that of the shaman, who drew his power from religious and supernatural forces. Like the minister and the priest, the physician has been looked to as a source of spiritual wisdom for guiding patients through the difficulties and stresses of critical periods in their lives, for providing relief from pain, and for helping to restore function and prolong life. Over hundreds of years, it has been expected that the patient who turns to a physician for help should play a dependent, obedient role with his doctor; and furthermore, that this doctor, in turn, should be available to his patient at all times for comfort, solace, wise, tender care, and the healing of sickness and wounds.

Lay people, certainly, and physicians themselves to some extent, have been aware that this relationship was an ideal not often fulfilled in the performance. As with ministers and priests,[2] there have been many physicians who were not capable of the wisdom, nobility of character, and discipline that their ideal roles demanded from their limited humanity. This human frailty has served as a frequent source of humor and dramatic caricature to novelists and playwrights, who have portrayed these idealized figures as vainly and pretentiously trying to fill up the empty spaces of their lofty roles with bluff and bluster. Nonetheless, this has been what patients have sought and hopefully expected from their physicians and what physicians have tried more or less successfully to fulfill in their work with their patients.

In order to play this magic helper role without too much conflict within his own personality, the physician himself has had to practice denial of his insecurity, of his fearfulness, of his lack of knowledge and feelings of inadequacy. For the busy physician there has always been so much to know and so little time to learn it all. He has had to compensate, or rather perhaps to overcompensate, for his feelings of uncertainty by appearing most certain himself, and by communicating certainty to the patient in a way that reinforces the feeling between himself and the patient that what is being done is proper. He has been dependent on continuous feedback from the patient that reassures and confirms his authority so that both he and the patient can feel security and safety in the treatment program.

In the early nineteenth century, or perhaps a little earlier, a new role began to develop for the physician in Western culture, one that gradually acquired more and more prestige, especially among the wealthy and the powerful. This new ideal evolved from an awakening reverence for the astonishing and rapidly developing technological sciences both in and outside of medicine. Unfortunately, scientific authority was associated with the fallacious oversimplification that the exclusive path to true knowledge lay through the elimination of emotional or spiritual involvement with the object of one's observation. The scientific ideal called for ruthlessly detached, uninvolved, neutral, painstaking attention to details in a search for lawful sequences and patterns. It had the advantage over the earlier idealization, of affording a more limited and more realistic point of view, less grandiose expectations for the patient, and detachment from a total involvement with gratification of the patient's needs on the doctor's part. The patient was, however, still supposed to be obedient, although not to the moral authority of wisdom and faith, but to the new scientific authority of technical abstract knowledge which would now serve as guide to ignorant emotional humanity.

However, in the past 40 or 50 yr., through psychoanalytic investigation, psychological studies, and social science research, there has been an increasing documentation of the effects of *authority* in medical practice. The authority of the physician in its own right plays a part in healing and relieving the patient's distress and disability, not only in terms of what is called the placebo effect, but also in terms of what is called the iatrogenic effect of reinforcing or contributing to the patient's distress and disability. Often the patient is the victim of the physician's investment, conscious or unconscious, in the caretaking relationship, which only increases the patient's sense of helplessness and dependency and spurs the physician on to try one thing after another. Sometimes it is the physician himself who is the victim of his own pseudoomnipotent responsibility who gives more and more time, attention, emotional investment, and even money to a patient who becomes increasingly demanding, frustrating, and unrewarding.

Balint et al. have described a particular relationship that can develop between primary physicians and their patients which illustrates a common pitfall of medical authority. It is characterized by a repetition of the same prescription—usually a mild sedative or psychotropic drug—over a period of many years. These long-repeat patients originally came complaining of unpleasant bodily sensations due to tensions and strains accumulating in the course of relatively unsatisfactory lives. Since they felt they needed "something," they went to their doctors to complain. Nothing in the way of localizable illness was found even after the most thorough clinical and laboratory investigations. The primary physician trained in illness-centered medicine could not achieve much, but he kept trying anyway—attested to by the high frequency of multiple diagnoses in this group. Gradually a strained relationship developed between the physician and the patient as the doctor tried harder and the patient remained unsatisfied. Finally a repeat prescription was introduced, and the relationship changed for the better. An insincere mutual appreciation based on an overevaluation of the drug and the physician replaced the strained unsuccessful effort.[3] Thus, we see the frustration and conflict that can develop in the obedient patient-scientific doctor type of authority relationship.

The contemporary world has given rise to a third medical model in which the patient is encouraged to be a partner and collaborator and to share the responsibility for his treatment with his physician. According to this new model, the physician no longer hides the name and nature of the treatment or medication that he provides for the patient. He calls medications by their generic names and discusses potential toxic properties as well as potential side effects (insofar as he can do so without provoking pseudo side effects by suggestion; he must guard against this by an appraisal of the patient's personality), and he shares with the patient the risks of other therapeutic interventions. The patient in this model questions the physician's authority, reads widely in popular medical literature, seeks consultation freely when in any doubt, and cooperates with his doctor as a mature, responsible partner in the enterprise of correcting whatever is ailing him. This role is broader but yet more realistic than the other authority role previously described. It explicitly states the limits of realistic expectations. Education and the mass media have played an important part in preparing patients for such collaboration. So has psychoanalysis.

The three models which have been delineated describe three varieties of physician: the wise healer, the skilled scientist, and the expert partner. These models all, to some degree, play a part in medical practice today, depending on the personal history and the personality of both patient and physician and upon the context in which patient and physician meet.

These three roles, which continue to be filled by primary physicians, are evident as well in psychiatric practice. There are many prevailing models in psychiatry today. One can still find the orthodox psychoanalyst sitting behind the patient where he cannot be seen, protecting his neutrality and anonymity, and watching carefully, like a scientist behind an instrument panel, manipulating regression and transference by the instrument of his verbal interpretation, treating the patient's illness with authoritative scientific skill. There is also the psychiatrist who acts out his notion of the big parent—alternating loving, kind, appreciative attention with scolding, yelling, and screaming at the patient to reeducate him toward health. However, the prevailing model in psychiatry today, especially in official psychiatry as it is taught in medical schools and institutes, is that of the partnership. Dependent relationships are regarded as naive and childish— perhaps necessary temporarily as a preparatory stage for a relationship of greater independence. The psychiatrist is here committed to the ideal of encouraging maturity, independence, and individual responsibility in his patients. Comfort, guidance, succor, and solace are considered to be temporary supportive measures and subordinate tactics to be used only when the severity of the patient's difficulties make them necessary. Dependent needs met by supportive techniques are viewed as transitory aspects of the transference relationship, manifestations to be "worked through."

Struggle against reductionism in medical education

The dominant trend in medical education, as well as in medical practice in this century, has been toward technical excellence at the expense of a more humanistic doctor-patient relationship. William James, in the nineteenth century, warned against the tendency toward materialistic reductionism in medicine wherein the problems of the whole person in his life situation would be oversimplified and reduced to the mechanics of the parts of his body. Adolf Meyer, later on, throughout his long career in this century, repeated the same warning and fought, sometimes successfully, against the tendency to make diagnoses by exclusion and to reduce problems of life conflicts and their manifestations to mere issues of anatomy and chemistry. In 1942, a popular book that went through many editions, by a professor of pediatrics, Dr. Aldrich, was entitled *Babies Are Human Beings*. Many years later another book to do with similar concerns appeared: *The Rights of Infants* by Margaret Ribble. We cite these works so as to lend some historic retrospectives to these struggles that for a long time have gone on against the increasing narrowing of tendencies in medical education and practice toward technical competence, proficiency, highly specialized knowledge, and detachment from the emotional aspects of the patient and his illness or injury. Pressures from the early Flexner report and the later establishment of specialty boards in medicine contributed to an increasing population of highly qualified specialists in narrow fields of medicine and surgery, successfully concentrating on eliminating infections, discovering the causes of hitherto obscure diseases, and devising innovations in surgery that would prolong life and minimize disability. The success of this technical scientific development and the skill and qualifications of this highly specialized population of physicians cannot be questioned. They have made enormous contributions, not only to America but to the population of the entire world, in prolonging life, minimizing or eliminating diseases of certain kinds, and preventing and compensating for disabilities that were not previously amenable to treatment.

Gradually, however, general practitioners who treat private patients and their families have become fewer and fewer in number until they have become a minority in medicine. They have also recently achieved their own specialty status and specialty board. With the unanticipated population explosion in this country following World War II we have not only a shortage of general practitioners, but a shortage of all doctors in all specialties. There has been a profusion of complaints about the impersonality, the unavailability, and the inadequate attention patients have experienced from the physicians they went to for help.[4]

With the increasing frequency of the problems resulting from the lack of attention to the emotional aspects of medical practice, medical societies and medical schools, residency training programs, and postgraduate continuing-education programs have turned to psychiatrists for help. They have asked psychiatrists to participate in designing educational programs to compensate for earlier educational deficiencies regarding emotional disorders. A World Health Organization report in 1961 called attention to the new role that psychiatry had begun to play in the overall teaching of medicine. This report emphasized the psychiatrist's holistic interest in human beings and in the social realities of the human context, as well as the increasing importance of the role of the psychiatrist in improving medical practice and medical education.[6]

Psychiatrists have not been fully prepared to assume this leadership.[7] Ideological differences and the struggles for power between psychoanalytic and psychiatric groups in this country and abroad have confused their medical colleagues. This has been especially evident in problems of language, wherein each ideological sect tends to develop its own vocabulary for formulating the problems of patients and methods of treatment, and promoting its own group by avoiding the vocabularies of other groups.[8] Attempts to present psychiatry in a theoretical system as a body of established and classified *facts* about causes and treatment of mental disease can only puzzle and repel the intelligent, well-educated, and sophisticated student, whereas the less critically minded student might be swayed by whatever fashion or dogma was most acceptable in his locality at any given time. It is understandable, then, that physicians are suspicious of the efforts of their psychiatric colleagues to teach them new skills. However, with proper humility and modesty much can be taught, at least tentatively[9] —for although a consensus on systematic theory is lacking, there is a sound body of pragmatic knowledge.

New demands on primary physicians

Over the past 20 or 30 yr. increasing attention has been paid to remedying the inadequacy of undergraduate training in psychiatry. Cope, a surgeon himself, has insisted on the importance of more study in the humanities and in the social sciences for medical students.[10]

There have also been efforts to provide practicing physicians with postgraduate education in psychiatry.[11-13] The National Institute of Health, the American Psychiatric Association, and the Academy of General Practice, among other groups, have been actively involved in this area. Conferences, colloquia, and joint committees have been established on national, regional, state, and local levels with the collaboration of medical societies, the Academy of General Practice, and the American Psychiatric Association. Last year the American Psychiatric Association published a task force report on psychiatric education and the primary physician. This report states:

> ... As currently conceived, the community mental health center will depend heavily upon the primary physician in the community—primary in the sense that he be the chief case-finder and the chief executive of preventive efforts at the family level. It also seems likely that the medical staff of most centers will include many physicians who are not psychiatrists, but who will need the kind of training that can be provided by postgraduate education programs in order to function best within the community mental health center.
>
> In similar fashion, state mental hospitals as well as many local and private hospitals already depend heavily upon family physicians for aftercare of patients upon discharge. . . . one obvious way to improve the communications between psychiatrists and family physician, and at the same time to give the family physician a firmer base for managing emotional concomitants in the illnesses of all his patients, is to involve him more meaningfully in the treatment and disposition medical personnel.[14] [Pp. 9–10.]

The quote above, and the one to follow, describe the expectations psychiatric organizations, and organizations representing general practitioners, have formulated for primary physicians. In 1966, a joint committee with representatives from the American Academy of General Practice and the American Medical Association, Section on General Practice, agreed on the following areas to be included in what they called the core content of family medicine. This consisted of two main aspects: clinical and sociological.

> I. *Clinical Aspect.* Within this category: 1) doctor-patient relationships, which covers such points as types of doctor-patient relationships (activity-passivity, guidance-cooperation, and mutual participation); role of illness in society (patient expectations and physician expectations); patient characteristics of all age groups, pre-natal, infancy, pre-school, school, adolescent, young adulthood, middle-age, older-age, and the dying (physical, cultural, and psychological); continuing care; physician participation; interview technique and setting; self-knowledge; technical skills; and attributes (consideration, compassion, interest, acceptance, empathy, responsibility, and flexibility).

Also included under clinical aspects: 2) preventive medicine, covering health education; normal growth and development; environmental influence; crisis information; and community relations; 3) diagnosis, including history; recognition of normal deviations; 4) treatment and management, including physical, mental, and environmental illnesses; chronic and debilitating illnesses; emergency care; family counseling; and terminal care; 5) techniques in diagnosis, therapy, and management covering such fields as psychiatry and psychology, pharmacology, preventive medicine, and behavioral sciences; 6) rehabilitation, including convalescent care and family adjustment; 7) consultation and referrals.

II. *Sociological Aspects.* Within this category are: 1) family and community, including sociology and the family group and related institutions; psychology of the person and group; ecology of the home and community; and religious beliefs, practices, and creeds; 2) community resources; and 3) allied and paramedical personnel.[14] [Pp. 9–10.]

We see what psychiatrists expect from the primary physicians in relation to community mental health centers and the aftercare of patients, and we see what the official governing bodies of the primary physicians themselves expect, and it all adds up to a very tall order indeed. The pendulum appears to have swung from an extreme of an ideal detachment to the opposite extreme of an ideal involvement in a broad range of emotional and social ills. Both extremes are equally unrealistic. One might anticipate that the response of physicians to these ideal expectations might be less than enthusiastic. Indeed, that seems to have been true. In a preliminary survey of the literature on this subject, done several years ago, we found that the percentage of physicians enrolled in postgraduate psychiatric education programs was generally not more than 10 percent of the primary physicians practicing in any specific area. More recently, in the course of the study we have just completed, we found an increase of up to 25 percent and more of the primary physician population who are participating in postgraduate psychiatric education. This remarkable increase in the psychiatric involvement of primary physicians must be credited to the individual and joint efforts of members and groups from the National Institutes of Health, the American Psychiatric Association, and the Academy of General Practice, who have been sponsoring continuing-education programs, and recruiting with greater insight and skill over the years.

Our research project was sponsored by the National Institutes of Health, whose representatives shared our conviction that it was important to gather data from physicians themselves concerning their needs, attitudes, practices, and interests with regard to psychiatric services and education.[17] It seemed clear that the ambitious programs that official psychiatry and official general medicine had designed for primary physicians were based on a dearth of information about the ways in which the primary physician deals with and what he feels about the psychiatric aspects of his practice. We believed that our research would be invaluable to these programs. By presenting them with reliable data about physicians, data that could be elaborated into further surveys and programs, the assumption that a homogeneous group of physicians with homogeneous needs existed would be challenged, so that a greater variety of programs could be offered to heterogeneous groups, who could participate on an equal level with their teachers in determining programs best suited to their particular needs and interests.[18]

Method

A self-administered questionnaire was distributed by mail to 3119 primary physicians representing the sum of nine distinct subsamples. The questionnaire contained 84 items and took approximately 20 min. to complete. The rate of return from the different subsamples varied from 80 percent to about 10 percent, depending upon the intensity of follow-up and the various resources for follow-up available. The overall return rate was 37 percent. The data from the questionnaire were coded, key punched, and verified. An IBM 360 computer provided the analytical printout. Various statistical and analytical operations were performed.

Five of the nine subsamples were hospital based, and four community based. The hospital samples were solicited from attending physicians on the staffs of five different hospitals, three of which were urban: a 400-bed hospital in Portland, Oregon; a 575-bed hospital in Manhattan, New York; and a 165-bed hospital in Queens, New York. The two other hospitals were suburban: a 300-bed hospital in Westchester County, New York, and a 458-bed hospital in New Hyde Park, New York.

The community-based subsamples were:

1. All the primary physicians in a geographically distinct urban area in Manhattan, New York, who completed and returned their questionnaire with no or minimal follow-up (the West Side catchment area).

2. The physicians in the same geographic area who completed their questionnaire later and only after intense telephone and personal follow-up procedures.

3. All the primary physicians in a geographically distinct mixed urban and suburban area around and including Philadelphia who completed and returned their questionnaires with no follow-up.

4. All the primary physicians in the same area around and including

Philadelphia who completed their questionnaires after a moderate amount of telephone follow-up.

Findings—Fused sample

First we shall describe the findings derived from the fusion of all nine subsamples and then compare these data with the results obtained from combining the two subsamples from the West Side catchment area in New York City.

Considering the diversity of geographic, ethnic, and other factors, the fact that very similar percentages and figures were obtained on most of the questionnaire items from all these subsamples leads us to believe that we can project a profile that might reliably characterize the physician in America today in urban and suburban areas in regard to certain issues.[19] About 25 percent of typical physicians would refuse more or less invariably to deal with emotional aspects of their medical or surgical practices. A greater proportion of general practitioners than specialists are interested and involved in these aspects of medicine. The major determining factor for whether or not the typical physician pays attention to emotional aspects of his practice is the extent to which such emotional factors interfere with the diagnosis and treatment of organic illnesses.

The first treatment choice for a typical physician when confronted with emotionally disturbed patients is to provide physical examination and reassurance. The second choice is to give opportunity for ventilation, and the third choice is advice. Drugs are listed fourth. The physician is very cautious in his use of drugs, naming more correct drugs for anxiety than for depression and even fewer for schizophrenia. More than a third of physicians refuse to deal with schizophrenia at all. Our findings contradict those of other surveys which report enormous quantities of prescriptions of minor tranquilizers; our survey suggests underutilization of psychotropic drugs as well as a high proportion of incorrect usage of these drugs. Physicians prescribe the minor tranquilizers in the general treatment of many physical illnesses; they may consider the use of these psychotropic drugs as part of overall medical treatment rather than as treatment of emotional problems in their practices.

The typical physician would prefer to refer patients who present emotional problems to other facilities for treatment rather than to treat these patients himself. However, about 20–30 percent of these physicians would be willing to try to help out if they were provided with adequate help and guidance. Although the typical physician claims that referrals are his main preference for treatment and disposition of emotional disorders in his practice, 31 percent of the doctors did not refer more than 2 patients in a 6-mo. period.[20] Is it that the typical physician is unable to recognize emotional problems, or does he not consider it his responsibility to refer patients who have these problems for help? It is interesting to note that there is a very high positive correlation between the degree of confidence the physician feels in diagnosing and in managing the emotional problems of his patients and the degree to which he seeks expert help with the management of disturbed patients and makes appropriate psychiatric referrals. In other words, the physician who feels most confident and secure in dealing with the emotional aspects of his practice is also the physician who makes the most use of psychiatric resources and education, whereas the physician who feels the least secure is the one who makes the least use of these facilities. This suggests that the mechanism of denial is being used. The physician who feels inadequate and insecure in the face of the emotional problems in his practice may tend to deny their existence. He fails to diagnose or treat these problems, does not refer psychiatric patients for treatment when indicated, and does not seek help in managing them.[21] Although most physicians complain of the inadequacy of community facilities, at the same time they utilize little of what is available.

West Side catchment area—The environment

Before we focus in greater depth on the physicians of the West Side catchment area in New York City, we shall first describe this area and its population. This is the upper West Side of Manhattan, roughly between Forty-second Street and Ninety-sixth Street. In the late 1930s to the mid-1950s this neighborhood consisted of brownstones and apartment houses housing mainly an upwardly mobile, lower-middle-class to upper-middle-class, Jewish population. Children played freely in the streets with their age mates from neighboring houses and apartments. There was less traffic and litter in those days, so children were able to play many different kinds of sports and ball games in the street. They also felt free to enjoy and explore Central Park and Riverside Park day and night. They often visited each other in their homes and apartments and listened to ball games and to the serial dramas on the radio before television came in. A typical neighborhood ritual was attending the Saturday matinee at a local movie theatre, where the children would go in groups of four or five without an adult tagging along, and eat popcorn, candy, and ice cream.

The stores in this neighborhood were open late. In the summertime people frequently sat out on chairs on the sidewalks, visiting, talking, and chatting with each other.

The average doctor in those days was a local family physician who was well known to the children as he passed them by, many of whom he himself had delivered, had cared for as they grew up, and whose families called on him for all their medical and many of their emotional needs. He made house visits, and his office was open to the people in the neighborhood for treatment of their cuts, scratches, infections, and injuries. He was definitely more of a wise old shaman than an objective scientific authority.

By 1955, this scene was undergoing a drastic change. Ralph Schoenstein has splendidly described his experiences growing up on West Seventy-eighth Street and returning to it as an adult in a novel, *A Block*. Traffic in the area had increased to such an extent that street games had become impossible and had disappeared. It was not only unpleasant but also unsafe to walk in the streets and parks at night because of the increasing amount of crime; there were muggings, assaults, purse snatchings, and other crimes. The increased crime rate was associated with the influx of the former ghetto population from the South moving into the ghettos of the North, and with the large numbers of poor, unskilled immigrants from Puerto Rico.

The single- and two-family brownstones were gradually converted into smaller units for multiple-family usage. Low-income and welfare cases were crowded into the small apartments that resulted from the conversion of the brownstones. Many homosexuals moved into the single-room-occupancy boardinghouses, hotels and rooming houses that had sprung up in this area. Increasing numbers of housing units became useless and obsolete, waiting to be torn down for urban renewal programs. The old movie theaters that the children had gone to for Saturday matinees disappeared, converted into TV studios or to supermarkets.

In the neighborhood itself, young families were beginning their exodus to the suburbs, leaving behind the older people. Many small retail stores and specialty shops were also moving out, either to the East Side or to the suburbs. The population of Manhattan as a whole declined, including that of this particular area. There was also a decrease in the number of jobs available in manufacturing and in retail trade throughout the entire city. Meanwhile there was an increase in the number of executive, financial, and industrial management jobs, and in the amount of office space. However, these high-paying jobs were mostly filled by people commuting to the city from the suburbs.

Hence, we note an overall decline in the neighborhood as a whole, in the quality of living, and in the socioeconomic level.

There have been a number of attempts at improvement in recent years. We have urban renewal programs, mostly middle income, in the Lincoln Center neighborhood, and mixed income in the upper 90s. In certain areas brownstones have been renovated and occupied by young professional people whose guests and visitors, nevertheless, need to be on the constant lookout for crime when they come to visit their friends. There also are renovated tenements and new luxury, middle-, and upper-income apartments. A few well-to-do and middle-income blocks exist in the area, with bars, restaurants, and stores that are oriented to a more racially integrated population. There is even, in some sections, an attempt at an upper Greenwich Village, with a Bohemian, artistic population taking advantage of the less expensive housing in this neighborhood, as compared with the East Side of the city. Little boutiques and craft shops are opening up, especially around Seventy-second Street. However, there remain many very deteriorated hotels, apartments, and rooming houses. There is still a large, hardcore, hopeless group of welfare and unemployed people living on very restricted incomes.

As elsewhere in the country, one sees here a deterioration of traditional family patterns, a restless and disturbed youth population, and an alarming increase in narcotic activities. A once popular children's play area on the West Side now has no children playing in it anymore; it is widely known as "Needle Park"! More children are staying out late or all night, their whereabouts unknown to their parents. There has been a great increase in aggressive, hostile, and destructive behavior in the schools, with vandalism occurring more often now in the earlier grades of elementary school. A large group of families is fatherless. In a considerable number of families the mother works, and adequate day-care facilities are lacking. There is an unusually and increasingly large pool of single, unattached adults whose social and psychological adjustment varies from good to marginal to decompensated.

A few years ago, a community survey described a representative family from this neighborhood: The father was alcoholic, unemployed, with incestuous impulses toward his daughter; the mother was depressed, hypochondriacal, and phobic; the paternal grandmother, who lived with the family in the small apartment, was senile, paranoid, diabetic, and arthritic; the oldest son, who lived from time to time in the same apartment, was delinquent and a school dropout; the daughter was an unwed mother with periodic fainting spells; the second son was a drug addict; the third son was a truant, failing in school, glue sniffing, and refusing to leave his room; the youngest was mentally retarded; a maternal uncle was in a state hospital diagnosed as a chronic schizophrenic with recurrent episodes. Professional services to this family were provided by: the New York City Department of Social Services, the youth division of the police department, the family court, the juvenile court, the visiting nurse service, the Bureau of Attendance and the Bureau of Child Guidance of the Board of Education, the New York State Department of Mental Hygiene, the Housing Authority, a succession of priests, and a local hospital. Overwhelming and melodramatic as it sounds, it is nevertheless true.

The Roosevelt Hospital contains the community mental health center for the West Side catchment area and has worked hard and successfully to develop programs for this area under the leadership of Drs. Harley Shands and Stuart Keill. In 1969, 41 different community mental health projects were offered in this area, 84 percent of which were operating outside of the hospital. Two neighborhood care teams work in the community, locating people who need help and providing a variety of services such as home treatment, group discussions, group therapy, consultation services to staffs of other agencies, referral services, and special projects for single-room-occupancy houses and hotels.

The Mental Health Center of Roosevelt Hospital operates several drug abuse programs: methadone maintenance, identification and treatment of drug-addicted adolescents, support for Alcoholics Anonymous, an alcoholism service offering a variety of in- and outpatient, group, and individual therapies, outpatient help for relatives, friends, and employers of alcoholics, and liaison services with other agencies. It also provides counseling, consultation, and help to 14 different educational institutions in this area, including five special half classes at two different schools for disturbed children with learning difficulties.

West Side catchment area—Physician population

Much of our information about the physicians in the West Side catchment area is based on material obtained from 34 interviews conducted in person or over the telephone with physicians selected randomly from this subsample, as well as from the results of the questionnaire survey. A return rate of 65 percent of the questionnaires was obtained after intensive telephone and personal follow-up.

The total physician population of this area has declined by 40 percent in the period of 6 yr. between 1964 and 1970. What are the physicians like who have remained in this neighborhood? In contrast to the physicians in the other subsamples, they are a much older and a much more lonely group.

Like many other older people who have stayed on in the neighborhood, these physicians feel more and more isolated and frightened in relation to the world around them. The children they delivered and took care of have grown up and left the city for the suburbs; so have their own children grown up and left. They work as solo practitioners as they always have, not as part of a group practice. They do not have much investment in hospitals, with which they have a peripheral association, if any at all. Many of them played active and even leading roles in the city hospitals 20, 30, or 40 yr. ago. Now they are more restricted by their age, infirmity, and other circumstances. Twenty years ago, they kept their waiting room doors open and people came in and out all day. Nowadays, they keep their waiting room doors locked and see their patients by appointment or after carefully identifying them through the peepholes.

In their practice of medicine, they attempt to keep up with the literature, and many of them—more than the national average—take courses in all branches of medicine, including psychiatry, to improve their skills, even while in their 70s and 80s. They are very cautious in prescribing medication or other forms of treatment, tending to rely on drugs and procedures familiar many years ago. They are reluctant to try new drugs, such as tranquilizers, or other psychotropics, or even antibiotics, until they have been on the market for a long time and have been adequately tested. Many of these physicians have long ago stopped prescribing amphetamines for obesity control because of the tendency to become deluged with requests from youngsters who are looking for kicks. One physician mentioned that he had put an extra lock over his door and taken his sign down because there were so many youngsters coming in from the street to ask for amphetamines. None of the physicians treated or had any interest in learning how to treat drug dependency problems of any kind or drug addiction, in spite of the high incidence of patients suffering from alcoholism and drug abuse in this area. Most of the primary physicians surveyed showed no awareness of the many facilities afforded them and their patients by the Community Mental Health Center. The primary physician was conspicuous by his absence; he had little or nothing to do with community mental health services and the families they served.

One of us taught a group of the physicians from this neighborhood in a postgraduate course given in psychiatry at Roosevelt Hospital. Thirteen physicians with an age range of 39 to 82 signed up. Most of them were in their middle to late 60s. Some were still married; some were widowers. They all expressed a poignant feeling of loneliness and distress at the changes that had taken place around them. They experienced considerable pleasure in the camaraderie of the course they were taking, and also in the seminars which some of them had been taking over a period of many years. The physicians were a warm, good-natured, appreciative, and very down-to-earth group who were more than ordinarily aware of the harmful effects of medical intervention in the form of drugs, advice, or surgery, particularly on the aged patients they were treating. Hence, the methods they preferred tended to be very conservative, with the emphasis on watching, waiting, and maintaining contact rather than prescribing or trying to cure in any immediate way. Exceptions were made for the standard types of ailments such as infections.

The median age is 59. There is a high percentage of Jewish physicians (73 percent) and a much larger proportion of foreign born (45 percent). Twenty percent of the physicians in the West Side of New York moved out of the neighborhood between 1968 and 1970, with very, very few moving in. There is also a high rate of death and retirement: 19 percent in the 2-yr. period between 1968 and 1970 in this West Side New York area.

The typical West Side physician has been in practice in the present location for over 20 yr., prescribes psychotropic drugs infrequently, and has a high incidence of patients suffering from alcoholism, adult behavior problems, and senility; he frequently recognizes emotional problems in his practice but infrequently uses either consultation, referral, postgraduate education, or any community facilities. He would like a screening service which would provide psychiatric evaluation, furnish a report of the findings and recommendations, and also return the patient to his primary physician. The preference for such a screening service was also true for the fused sample.

Most of the physicians are not willing to see patients for aftercare, even with help. These physicians in the West Side of New York make fewer referrals than the rest of the samples; they use fewer psychiatrists when referring, and 34 percent complain that they rarely or never were able to find psychiatrists for emergencies. Fifty percent of the physicians frequently or usually found their patients resistant to psychiatric referrals. They felt less need for help with the emotional problems of their patients (64 percent), and only about 19 percent actually stated that they treat emotional difficulties of patients in their practice.

Where are the younger doctors in New York City? They are moving into positions as staff physicians in the teaching hospitals, joining medical groups, migrating to the suburbs, opening offices on the wealthier East Side or in the new luxury apartment buildings on the West Side. Those younger doctors who have a part-time private practice or group practice will often also have a part-time or full-time job in a prestige teaching hospital. Many will treat ghetto patients from the catchment area under Medicare and Medicaid on a salary basis in the emergency rooms, clinics, and inpatient services of the hospital, while in their private offices they will see wealthier patients.

There was one young physician we interviewed who had settled in the West Side area by choice and set up a general practice there. When asked why he had decided on this unfortunate area, he said that it was because he wanted to work with a more ethnically varied practice and did not like the affluent, prestige atmosphere of a university hospital or of the East Side neighborhood. He had been trained in a foreign medical school and enjoyed an interesting social life with people who were mostly in the theater and television industry and who resided in the more well-to-do apartments on the West Side. His practice consisted mostly of middle-class patients who came from his social contacts, but it also included a large percentage of middle-class black and Puerto Rican patients. He did not accept Medicaid patients, refusing to devote time to the required paper work.

We can say from the results of our study that the attitude toward psychiatry among these younger doctors is even more cautious and more reserved than among the older physicians working in the West Side neighborhood. A typical response from a younger, highly specialized doctor would be, "You wouldn't want a dermatologist to treat a gastric ulcer, would you?" However, in certain specialty groups, especially the nonsurgical ones, there is a much greater sensitivity to and use of psychiatric resources in terms of consultation and referral, as well as in use of the community agencies.

We shall now be quoting from sample interviews that we had with various physicians in the neighborhood to give a more direct and immediate focus to the material that has been presented in this paper. Each of the three physicians we are going to quote at some length is representative of the group and is in the 60s or 70s.

> *Physician 1.* Ninety percent of my patients now come in with psychosomatic complaints. They are all in the older age range. When I first started my practice, they were all younger people who came in with actual medical complaints, teen-agers, people in their 20s and 30s. They were never asking for sleeping pills or pep pills.
>
> Many people than complained of bronchitis, sore throats, or infections—not today, even with the increased air pollution. There is much less respiratory illness complained of. . . .
>
> The traffic in the street now is terrible—buses, trucks, cars, and noise. This continues to 1:00 A.M. and starts at 4:00 A.M. . . . patients of mine—older people

who live in this building—complain of teen-agers and young men and even young girls who knock them down, particularly the old ladies. They knock these old ladies down and search them for any money they can find, looking in their brassieres, stocking, and panties as well as their purses, and then escape by running away to the park. They do it also on the buses, and the bus driver ignores it and is afraid to do anything about it.

Physician 2. I moved here in the mid-1940s because I had two young children and this was a very desirable neighborhood then. I moved here for their sake more than 25 yr. ago. I did general practice, which I still do although I have my boards in internal medicine now. I see patients only by appointment referred by other doctors or other patients.

There has been no great change in my practice although most of my patients who used to live here have moved away, but they still come to see me here from Westchester and Long Island. The biggest change in my practice is the enormous amount of time spent with and the interference from various medical insurance plans—private and government. I may spend 3 to 4 hr. after office hours on paper work. . . . The expenses of running an office in rent, salary, and other upkeep costs have soared enormously. It soon won't be possible for a solo practitioner to keep up an adequately equipped office no matter what his fees are. . . . I make house calls only for great emergencies now. It is too hazardous, expensive, and difficult to park and travel about late at night. . . . There are more acknowledged cases of emotional illness now. Perhaps they were denied or not noticed so much before. Patients are more enlightened now and speak more easily about their emotional conflicts, sexual problems, and other feelings.

I don't make new friends any longer. I do see my old friends who are still alive. I have no time for community activities, but I do see hope for the future. At one time I thought this whole neighborhood had become a vast slum. But now I see neighborhood block associations being formed by people who care about keeping their street clean and rejuvenating the appearance of the houses. Something can be done if people will do it.

However, it is still a very dangerous and violent area to an extent undreamed of 10 yr. ago. People are mugged very frequently. All of my patients who live in this area have been mugged at least once. One of my patients was mugged twice in one week. It is particularly disabling for men, who feel an enduring rage and helplessness after the mugging that is hard for them to deal with. They feel they should have done something.

The traffic is also dangerous. I would shudder to think of what would happen to children playing on these streets now.

My children grew up and went to school here and are now doing graduate work in Illinois and California. They will never come back to New York except for an occasional visit with us.

I regret not leaving New York years ago. I would have been much happier in a smaller, cleaner, and quieter town. I don't like the changes I see taking place in New York.

Physician 3. I would like to move, but I can't. My wife and I can't get around like we used to. I am trapped here. She is not well; I am not well; I am 73 yr. old. . . . .

I don't take Medicare or Medicaid patients. I send them to someone else or to the hospital or clinic. I make sure they get good care, but I won't accept them.

I can't handle the paper work, the bookkeeping, and the forms. You need a special course just to keep up with the nomenclature.

No, I don't see any Puerto Ricans or blacks, not in my private practice. It is not that I won't accept them; they won't call, except for drug addicts who ring your bell or knock on your door. I don't have anything to do with them.

No, there is not much new in my practice or treatments except some new drugs. There are new ones coming out all the time. Most of them don't amount to anything. Some are good. I have a much older practice now—mostly chronic cases of arteriosclerosis, heart disease, chronic emphysema, nephritis, arthritis. At the city hospital where I work, I see thousands of blacks and Puerto Ricans getting enormous amounts of medical attention. They get hundreds of dollars spent by the city on all kinds of tests they don't really need. They have no place to go, no money, so they come to the hospital for an outing and see their friends there. It is cool in the summer, it is warm in the winter; they sit there all day. They have machines for drinks, sandwiches, ice cream, and potato chips. They sit there and eat and talk and bring their children to play. . . .

Yes, the neighborhood change here is tremendous, unbelievable! Nothing is open anymore late at night. People are afraid to go out at night. You can't find a drugstore to fill a prescription anymore. It is getting worse and worse.

From these touching quotations, we see that a group of doctors, older than average, more individualistic, and more cautious than many others, experience their urban environment much as do their nonphysician friends and neighbors. Even though they are more frightened and isolated than their suburban colleagues, they do not differ very much in their attitudes and practices vis-a-vis the psychiatric aspects of their everyday work. Less than the younger physicians, less than the highly specialized university-based physicians, they still predominantly choose to avoid engagement with these problems.

Summary

Physicians today as well as in the past operate mostly within the model relationship of obedient patient to scientific authority. Some older physicians still take on the moral authority of the ancient religious models in preaching, lecturing, and advising their patients on the conduct of their lives. These authoritarian relationships, especially the narrow scientist-patient one, characterize the predominant and traditional form of doctor-patient relationship among specialists as well as general practitioners. It is this narrowly scientific relationship, reinforced by current medical education, that seems most responsible for the restricted nature of medical practice, with its defensive rejection of attention to the emotional problems of patients seeking help. It is this authoritarian, limited, scientific attitude that appears to stand in the way of a more comprehensive, more humane, and more flexible approach to the holistic treatment of patients, especially in the violent and difficult complexity of the present urban situation. The contemporary model of partnership and collaboration exists at present only in a growing minority of the younger doctors from the more advanced medical training centers.

We presented results of a large survey of physicians' attitudes and practices with psychiatric patients, services, and education. A more detailed description of a particular geographic urban area and its physician population was then compared with the larger sample to illustrate some of the problems with which physicians must cope today. The overwhelming majority of physicians in all the subsamples of the study want some kind of help in dealing with the emotional problems of their patients. The majority prefer some kind of consultation service that would evaluate the patient psychiatrically and send him back to his primary physician with a diagnosis and recommendations.

Appropriate consultation and educational services geared to the diverse variety of primary physicians should be further encouraged. Continued funding from private and governmental sources is essential.[22] Thus, these physicians could be helped to be more flexible in resolving the role conflicts they experience, and more understanding of their own personalities and of the needs of their patients, and of the social context in which they live.[23] Psychiatric education and services must allow for a broad range of doctor-patient relationships according to the personality requirements of both parties, in which doctors can function in their own unique styles and yet serve the best interests of patients and the community. There is no one model, no one role, no one way that is perfectly suitable for every doctor or for every patient.

References

1. Zabarenko, L., Pittenger, R. A., and Zabarenko, R. M.: Primary Medical Practice; A Psychiatric Evaluation. St. Louis, Warren H. Green, 1968.
2. Bentz, W.: Consensus between role expectation and role behavior among ministers. Community Ment. Health J. 4:391–306, 1968.
3. Balint, M., Hunt, J., Joyce, D., Marinker, M., and Woodcock, J.: Treatment or Diagnosis; A Study of Repeat Prescriptions in General Practice. London, Tavistock Publications, 1970.
4. Willer, D.: Palo Alto Times, Oct. 24, 1968.

5. Lipowski, Z. J.: Psychosocial aspects of disease. Ann. Int. Med. 71:1197–1206, 1969.
6. World Health Organization: Undergraduate Teaching of Psychiatry and Mental Health Promotion. World Health Org. Tech. Rep. Ser., 208, 1961.
7. Group for Advancement of Psychiatry: Medical Practice and Psychiatry: The Impact of Changing Demands, Report 7 # 58, 1964.
8. Brodsky, C.: A social view of the psychiatric consultation: The medical view and the social view. Psychosomatics 8:61–68, 1967.
9. Shepherd, M.: Psychiatric Education: General Review and Future Needs. Psychiatric Education. In: Davies, D. L., and Shepherd, M.: London, Pitman Medical Publishing Co., 1964.
10. Cope, O.: Man, Mind, and Medicine; the Doctor's Education. Philadelphia, J. B. Lippincott Co., 1968.
11. Brach, C. H. H.: Psychiatric training and the general practioner. Amer. J. Psychiat. 122:485–489, 1965.
12. De Boer, R. A., Jaspars, M. M. F., van Leeuven, P., van der Meer, F., Radder, J. J., and van Schaik, C. T.: An evaluation of long-term seminars in psychiatry for family physicians. Psychiatry, 33:468–482, 1970.
13. Balint, M.: The Doctor, His Patient, and the Illness. New York, International Universities Press, 1959.
14. Psychiatric Education and the Primary Physician, Task Force Report 2. Washington, D.C., American Psychiatric Association, 1970.
15. Coffey, E. M. Jr., Galbrecht, C. R., and Klett, C. J.: Brief hospitalization and aftercare in the treatment of schizophrenia. Arch. Gen. Psych. (Chicago) 24: 81–87, 1971.
16. Ehrenwald, J.: The general practitioner in community psychiatry: A progress report. In: Psychiatry in Medicine, Vol. 1, No. 3. Westport, Conn., Greenwood Periodicals, 1970.
17. Green, M. R., Haar, E., Hyams, L., and Philpot, J.: Physicians' interest and needs for psychiatric resources. New York J. Med. 71:1549–1552, 1971.
18. Green, M. R., Hyams, L., and Haar, E.: Interactional problems between mental health professionals and non-psychiatric physicians. Ment. Hyg. 55:206–213, 1971.
19. Pearson, J. B., and Bloom, B. L.: Report of a Survey of Colorado Medical Society Membership Initiated by the Colorado Mental Health Steering Committee. Boulder, Colo., Western Interstate Commission for Higher Education, August, 1969.
20. Hyams, L., Green, M. R., Haar, E., Philpot, J., and Meier, K.: Varied needs of primary physicians for psychiatric resources, (1. Behavioral indices). Psychosomatics 12:36–45, 1971.
21. Haar, E., Green, M. R., Hyams, L., and Jaffe, J.: Varied needs of primary physicians for psychiatric resources (II. Subjective factors). Psychosomatics. In press.
22. Borus, J. F.: The community mental health center and the private medical practitioner: A first step. Psychiatry 34:274–289, 1971.
23. Brodsky, C. M.: Decision making and role shifts as they affect the consultation interface. Arch. Gen. Psychiat. (Chicago) 23:559–565, 1970.

Discussion by Leston L. Havens, M.D., and Susan E. Miller, R.N.

Everyone is concerned about the primary physician; he is all but on the emergency list. At best, most seem discouraged about him. The primary physicians in this study are themselves discouraged. Most of those to whom the questionnaires were circulated did not even bother to return it, perhaps because they already have so much paper work to do. The authors seem discouraged, too. Actual suggestions as to what to do are taken up only in the last brief paragraph of this long report.

In fact, many of the patients concerned are passing out of the hands of the primary physician, into the hands of hospitals, emergency rooms, nurse practitioners, community mental health centers, catchment area facilities of many kinds, barely listed here. Although one aim of the report is to discuss the relationship of the primary physician to psychiatrists and psychiatry, almost nothing is said in detail about the specific relationships of the primary physician to places where most psychiatry and most psychiatrists are.

The bulk of paper is divided into four sections—one historical (the longest), one official (suggestions of various governing bodies as to what G.P.s need to know), statistical (conclusions of the material that was returned), and finally anecdotal. The whole input of the study is *ironical,* in the lowest key possible.

We are given a long-range survey of doctors' roles. Plainly the authors feel progress has been made in reaching toward collaborative functions. But as soon as we hear what actual practice is like on the West Side of New York City, the irony emerges. The West Side doctors have had to lock their doors, restrict their visiting hours, suspect the patients, hardly venture out. No conditions exist there remotely likely to make collaborative medicine possible.

In that light, the official statements are also ironical. We are told practitioners should know about doctor/patient relationships, consultation referral, and rehabilitation. What would the Council on Medical Education suggest the doctors do about their relationships with patients who steal their medicines or mug them on the street? How handle referrals when referral communication in great cities suggests signaling across outer space? And rehabilitation! How develop long-term rehabilitation plans when patients move yearly, step from agency to agency, and when the problems involve not just the patient, but father, mother, siblings et al., many of whom prove worse than the patient? These West Side doctors could write the black book of medical education.

And there is the irony of the statistical section. The plain fact is very few returned the questionnaire at all and, to some unstated extent, only after extra prodding. So removed were the practitioners from the investigative concerns that these concerns could hardly be investigated. What were the practitioners thinking and feeling? Certainly they are overworked (especially relative to contemporary standards of leisure), probably tired and discouraged. How many other forms had they been sent, how many projects, institutions, programs asked to contribute to without remuneration, often without thanks, just because they made the mistake of opening their morning mail? Or perhaps they felt, here was another government-sponsored form, another sign of the modern world so mechanical, impersonal, rapidly shifting and changing, deeply inimical to the idea of family practice. The irony is that the study itself may represent the very conditions which make the life of the primary physician perhaps impossible.

Why was the study so largely dependent on questionnaires? Or being done that way, why was no larger effort made to investigate the more than 60 percent who never responded? The size of that percentage not only throws all the findings into question; it raises an issue perhaps really pressing for investigation: who and how are these unresponsive but "primary" physicians, so tired, so angry, so indifferent, so what?

A series of ironies are presented—the impossibility of the collaborative model in the modern city, the irony of official expectations vs. actuality, the irony of a method of investigation representing the very world perhaps dooming the family practitioner, at least the family practitioner without two secretaries and four assistants.

We suspect the authors could have given us a still more poignant and touching document if these ironies had been exploited—so that we might all sense deeply how difficult the great ideals of general practice have become in the modern mechanized, computerized, crowded, and changing world.

part 5
RESEARCH IN THERAPY

Need Good Research
Destroy Good Therapy?*

CHARLES CLAY DAHLBERG, M.D.
JOSEPH JAFFE, M.D.

This chapter grows out of the experiences of a project in which we gave small doses of LSD to patients in analysis.[1] All the clinical work was done by one analyst (CCD) but there were an ex-practicing analyst (JJ), three psychologists, and a number of technicians on the team. The therapy sessions were audiotaped; 100-min. drug sessions and an active as well as an inactive placebo were used. Also, the experiment itself lasted over a period of from 16 to 22 mo. with each patient. We were interested in looking into clinical and psycholinguistic elements of the interaction as affected by LSD as opposed to the two placebos. The details of the design and findings, reported elsewhere, are not relevant to this paper. Here we are interested in certain ethical and procedural problems which relate to research in a psychoanalytic setting as we have encountered them.

* Joint project of the William Alanson White Institute and the Department of Communication Sciences, New York State Psychiatric Institute. Supported in part by National Institute of Mental Health grant number MH-11670 and the Department of Mental Hygiene, New York State.

Deception versus openness

Psychoanalysis is based upon truth, honesty, and openness. Double-blind procedures are based upon deception. We wished to give our patients LSD and they all agreed to this. However, we also wished to use each patient as his own control since we were limited to a small number of patients. Therefore, we also included an inactive placebo and, in an attempt to mimic some of the LSD effects, we also gave a stimulant drug, dextroamphetamine (DA). The analyst involved saw no problem in this until the time of the site visit. At this conference visitors from NIMH arrived to evaluate the proposal prior to its approval; the therapist was kindly asked to leave the room when the schedule of drugs was being planned. It suddenly dawned upon him that not only would he not know when a particular drug was being given but he was not going to be able to tell his patients that they were also getting amphetamine and a placebo. Certainly there could be little objection to an inactive placebo but he was also administering an active drug. In other words, he was telling them the truth but not the whole truth. Not only that, but dextroamphetamine is not innocuous.

After considerable soul searching the therapist managed to convince himself that he was not harming his patients; thereupon he devised a medical questionnaire, designed to get information about contraindications to amphetamine (such as hypertension), by asking a number of relevant as well as irrelevant questions which would obscure the purpose of the questionnaire (see Appendix A).

Deception, if employed, should be effective. The therapist was deceived not about what drugs were being given but about when they were being given. He told his patients that they would be given varying small doses of LSD. Following the end of the experiment a searching interview was conducted in which patients were asked among other things whether they thought they had been given another drug. Despite the fact that during the course of the therapy a number of patients said that they felt as though they were on "pep pills," none of them actually *believed* that they had been given any drug other than LSD.

After the interview they were told about the design of the project, how they had been deceived, and what we had found to date. One patient was mildly annoyed that he had been deceived, feeling he had paid for something he had not gotten. In truth, he had not paid for anything but psychotherapy and he agreed that this was true and then dropped the whole subject. Of the other 6, none resented having been deceived and 1 even expressed her admiration at the cleverness of the design.

Privacy and confidentiality versus transcription

Enough studies have been done on recording psychotherapeutic interviews to establish that with most patients, if this is an issue it becomes one only when the therapist himself is bothered by it.[2] This therapist rapidly realized that if he was going to tape 700 interviews to which other people would listen, he would have to get used to living in a goldfish bowl, and he did so.

These sessions were not merely taped. They were also transcribed, word for word, by six people. First we obtained a release not only for the administration of LSD but for audiotape recording. Then we coded all names, places, and anything else which might identify the patients. Third, we mixed up the sequence of the interviews so that a given transcriber would neither get tapes in the proper order nor get all of any one patient's sessions. We also instructed the patients to use first names when talking about other people and to do this whether or not they were being recorded. They practiced this long before they started having interviews taped. All of this worked fairly well; however, the fact is that the transcribers soon learned to identify patients by the sound of their voices, and they developed likes and dislikes for particular patients, largely based upon whether they spoke clearly or not. We believe that we have been able to establish an ethical sense in our transcribers and that they respect the privacy of the patients. Most likely the most important factor in cutting down inordinate curiosity in our transcribers is that transcribing somebody else's psycho-analysis is unutterably boring. It turned out that they couldn't care less about what the patient was doing after a few dozen hours of transcribing. What was lively to the analyst and to the patient who are actually involved was incredibly dull to a listener.

To ensure accuracy, transcriptions were relistened to and proofread; this turned up such incongruities in the transcriptions as "Aunt Liz" for "analyst" and "youth in Asia" for "euthanasia," which seemed to prove that our transcribers had a limited interest in content.

On the whole the patients did not seem to be concerned about the recording. On one occasion when the analyst forgot to turn on the tape recorder the patient reminded him that he hadn't heard the telltale click, and on another occasion when the patient had something to say after the tape recorder was turned off, she asked him to turn it on again so that they could get all of it on the record. The only time when it seemed that the recording procedure might have had some gross effect was once when a patient lowered his voice while discussing a matter which might have legal complications. Even he chuckled at that. In our retrospective interviews, all patients said that they did not think they held anything back because of the recording. Obviously this says nothing about the unconscious processes which might have been involved but we are convinced that they existed minimally if at all.

Physician responsibility versus double blind

Unlike many psychopharmacological projects where the observer is not responsible for patient care, in this project the observer was also the patient's doctor and was responsible for controlling the dose of the drugs that were given. He was also one of the blind men in the double blind.[3,4] It took many hours to hammer this one out and we finally did so in the following fashion. After each experimental session the analyst was required to answer two questions: (1) If the patient received LSD his next dose should be————, (2) If the patient received DA his next dose should be ————.

Since the analyst was not sure which drug had been given or what the dose had been he could only answer in terms of a specified increase or decrease. The instruction for the *correct* guess was followed. This system worked out well and allowed for the use of clinical judgment without breaking the code.

Individualism versus team cooperation

This was a long project. We have had nothing to report for 6 yr. The reason for this is that no data could be available until some time after all patients were run. A project of this kind needs the kind of personality that can tolerate frustration and delay. Each patient had 22 drug sessions at approximately 3- to 4-wk. intervals. One thing we did was find a few faintly related issues on which to report. It is no criticism to state that if you can't stand this kind of heat you shouldn't get into this kitchen.

As a team, we rapidly discovered even before we started our first patient that regular conferences were an absolute necessity. We obviously had many problems to think out in advance and we met once or more each week. We also started 1 patient first to see if our design worked and ran her for 3 mo. before starting any others. These conferences were of special importance in the interaction of two disciplines (psychoanalysis and psychology). Roles quickly became defined. The psychologist was trying to make as many observations as possible. The therapist was trying to keep his therapy as pure as possible. Only by hammering this out over many months were we able to achieve effective compromises, and we believe that the therapy was in fact not harmed nor was rigor of the research excessively watered down. These conferences continued with increasing frequency as results started coming in.

While working out the design we welcomed outsiders and visiting firemen. These were not only people from our funding organization but also interested colleagues from around the country. This kind of formal and informal research consultation proved invaluable. We received the most valuable help from the specialists at NIMH itself.

Modifications due to unforeseen event

We were well into the project when the first reports of chromosome damage from LSD appeared in the literature. Fortunately, we had a good working system by this time and could make the necessary adjustments to this news. The patients were in good rapport with the therapist and all agreed to continue with the experiment as we made arrangements with the Cyto-genetic Laboratory at the New York State Psychiatric Institute to start chromosomal studies. Such modifications of experiments must be rare but they do occur and in this case we were able to manage to continue without any real change in the study.

Interdisciplinary pressure and support

On a number of the issues in the experiment (deception, double blind, privacy) the therapist was under pressure to modify his customary procedures. Furthermore, he had initiated the experiment and had a great emotional investment in its success. There was never any question that he, as the therapist who had to deal with his patients, was the ultimate authority as to what would be done with them. He reported what was going on with them at the regular conferences, insofar as what was going on seemed related to the project, and he was given unqualified support by all team members. He in turn made every effort to assist the rest of the project members in getting any information they needed.

Specifically these are the ways in which we modified the psychotherapy in our experiment (for details see Appendix B).

1. The overall experimental context.
2. Two-hour psychotherapeutic sessions: at single-session fee.
3. Drug administration (double blind).
4. Scheduled pretherapy waiting periods.
5. Therapist presence during waiting periods.

6. Two pretherapy monologue recordings.

7. Regular paper-and-pencil tests.

8. Tape recordings of psychotherapeutic sessions.

9. Accompaniment of patient by attendant for 12 hr. after each drug session.

Under these circumstances, how was it that there were never any accusations of "pulling rank," or any serious conflict about goals? This question goes to the heart of the psychodynamics of interdisciplinary teams, which are not unlike families, and is much too long a story for this paper. But in a nutshell, the following points are relevant: "Rank" is diffused in a large system of truly interdependent elements. The key elements of this project were the 7 patients, the authors of this paper (one responsible for the therapy and the other for the psycholinguistic approach), a research psychologist with important supporting personnel who handled the data processing and statistical analysis, and, finally, the National Institute of Mental Health, which supported all the above and monitored the progress. The fact is that an uncooperative withdrawal of any of these key elements would have severely sabotaged or prematurely terminated the project. The therapeutic requirements (both for analyzing the patients and for comprehending the data) were too unique, the data-processing requirements were too specialized and monumental, and the statistical analyses too intricate and innovative to even imagine a respectable outcome of the project in the presence of severe interdisciplinary conflict. So much for the constraints. Of equal importance was the fact that most of the team had been psychoanalyzed and respected the therapist-patient relationship. All were committed to the concept of the experiment and none was so convinced of his omniscience (out of ignorance or insecurity) as not to expect to learn from the project. In addition, they all had other interests and so were not completely dependent upon either the project itself or any one aspect of it. The therapist had his independent practice and teaching duties. The psycholinguist had other psycholinguistic projects going. The research assistant was in love.

Related issues

It is frequently said that all the patient owes his analyst is to pay his fee and to free-associate. It is clear in this case our patients owed more than that. It was to be a long experiment and they were required to commit themselves to it, barring unforeseen events. All started on their own free will and some with eagerness. Since the analyst was to some degree dependent upon them for his project, this could force countertransference problems, so it became necessary to exclude subjects who seemed likely to be uncooperative because of excessive passive-aggressive tendencies.

Transference problems were exemplified by the following: One of the ways in which we forced commitment for the long-term stay on the patient was by the use of a release. This release was for the use of LSD and recordings and was legalistically phrased (see Appendix C). Patients were asked to have it witnessed by a family member if possible and also to discuss it with their lawyer or any person they desired. Several purposes were served by this document: (1) It ensured informed consent. (2) It was evidence of our seriousness and so probably convinced the patients that they had to be serious about their commitment. But this was not completely salutory inasmuch as many patients had the feeling at the beginning of the experiment that they were suddenly less important to the analyst than the experiment was. This feeling never seemed to last long since it apparently was not true in any individual case. One patient, however, said following the experiment that she felt that the experiment itself had done a remarkable amount of good because for the first time it forced her to take *herself* seriously. This sort of attitude is more of a problem for an outcome study than for a process study as ours was.

The question may be asked whether the setting as we have described it promotes regression and immaturity. There are many reasons to think that this might be true. Certainly the sessions are longer, there is the baby-sitting of the attendant with the patient, and many other things. However, it does not seem that this regression and immaturity occurred and we think the reason is simply that the analyst did not encourage it. Also, the patients were given tasks and responsibilities over the course of the experimental day. These were two recorded monologues which they were required to produce and a 30-min. paper-and-pencil test at the end of the 2-hr. psychotherapy session. Perhaps most important was that patients were implicitly encouraged to recognize the fact that they were part of a collaborative project.

Can an analyst remain objective when he has needs and goals beyond the analysis? There is no doubt that in this case there was a strong need for all members of the team to do as good a job on the research as possible. This was probably even more true for the analyst, who was not only the principal investigator but a highly visible subject occupying a unique position. This never became a real problem. The case never arose where there was a conflict between the needs of the research and the needs of the patient, and if such a conflict had arisen it undoubtedly would have been resolved in favor of the patient. The fact that no such conflict arose probably was due to the fact of the aforementioned careful planning and mutual support.

Patients felt special when they were brought into the experiment. It has also been mentioned that they felt the experiment was more special than they were. Does the patient feel rejected when the project is over and he no longer is so special? Perhaps it's a function of a long experiment that specialness wears off and tedium replaces it. Most patients enjoyed the LSD and most enjoyed their special status. They reported cocktail party conversations they had had about it, and some of these stories even came back to the analyst through third parties. However, everything becomes old hat sooner or later and most of the patients were relieved when the experiment was over and some of the more tiresome aspects of the project could be dropped.

An element of the collaboration between patient and analyst was that each gave the other something beyond the usual. The patient offered extra time and his extended cooperation. The analyst also offered extra time in the second hour of the experimental day (paid for by the project and not the patient) and LSD psychotherapy itself. We like to think that this tit for tat helped diminish excessive dependency, increased the sense of collaboration, and except on a transferential level gave the patients no reason to think they got something special because they were fascinating, which they were only in this context. In fact most patients do not think they are so fascinating. Their self-esteem is generally so low that they are much more concerned about being boring than fascinating.

Patients were also told that there was no assurance that LSD would help them. If we knew how LSD affected communication in psychotherapy, we wouldn't have to do an experiment. This was convincing. However, there was no denying that the analyst thought the drug could be useful to some people or else he wouldn't be doing all this work. It was also quite clear that not enough work had been done so that anyone could identify the mechanism even if it were, in fact, useful to some persons. The main emphasis was consequently an attempt to find out what happens to the dyad, clinically and psycholinguistically, when patients took drugs under controlled circumstances. With these sophisticated patients, this goal was easily understandable. They all knew that many drugs worked but that we did not know exactly how they worked. In effect the patients consented to be guinea pigs, hoping they would be helped, feeling part of something important, a little glamorous, and having confidence that there was little chance of any harm. We were interested in process, they in outcome. These disparate goals need not be disjunctive.

Summary

In summary, our conclusion is that good research *need* not destroy good therapy, but taken uncritically, this statement can be misleading. Good research increasingly requires complex procedures, large interdisciplinary teams, generous outside support, and the understanding of systems larger than the dyadic relationship or the family. Thus we should qualify the conclusion to require *certain kinds* of therapists and *certain kinds* of researchers.

References

1. Jaffe, J., Dahlberg, C. C., and Feldstein, S.: Practical aspects of systematic research in psychoanalytic office settings: Report of the committee on research. *In:* Masserman, J. H. (Ed.): The Ego, Vol. XI of Science and Psychoanalysis, New York, Grune & Stratton, 1967, pp. 202–222.
2. Haggard, E. A., Hiken, J. R., and Isaacs, K. S.: Some effects of recording and filming on the psychotherapeutic process. Psychiatry 28:169–191, 1965.
3. Cole, J. O.: Peeking through the double blind. *In:* Efron, D. H. (Ed.): The Proceedings of the Sixth Annual Meeting of the American College of Neuropsychopharmacology, San Juan, Puerto Rico, 1967, pp. 979–84.
4. Tétreault, L., and Bordeleau, J.: On the usefulness of the placebo and of the double-blind technique in the evaluation of psychotropic drugs. Psychopharmacol. Bull. 7:44, 1971.

Appendix A

Medical History Questionnaire

Have you ever had eczema, asthma, hay fever, high blood pressure, heart disease, liver or kidney ailments, diabetes, chronic eye disease, tuberculosis, epilepsy? If "yes," underline and give details.

Have you ever taken any of the following drugs: digitalis, morphine, Dexedrine, Benzedrine, Thorazine, ergotamine, Serpasil, nitroglycerine, Tedral, epinephrine? If "yes," underline and give details.

Have you ever had an unusual or adverse reaction to any drug or food? If "yes," give details.

Appendix B

Some Details of Therapy Modification

The patient came to the analyst's office at 1:00 P.M. and left at about 6:00 P.M. in the company of an attendant who remained in his home until the next morning. He was urged to stay at home that evening and discouraged from having visitors or telephoning. In a sense he was hospitalized for a day. The following remarks deal with those modifications of analytic technique not dealt with previously.

After the first few placebo sessions some rankled at the enforced seclusion. One compulsive worker rejoiced that she was able to be idle without guilt. This was therapeutic if only temporarily.

The modifications of the usual technique produced by the extended session can be controlled in part by extended placebo sessions but not for the patient who has trouble getting through 50 min. productively to begin with. Those who want a longer time are getting a gift. Their pay is their service as an experimental subject. We think this message got across.

The pretherapy waiting periods offered a special problem. They were necessary because the drug takes time to reach full effect, but because of patient apprehension and the special nature of LSD, patients couldn't be left alone. So the therapist stayed with them during this waiting period until he was sure they had had LSD two times. This usually meant about six times in all (two LSD plus two placebo plus two amphetamines). The patients called it babysitting. The therapist wrote, read, politely discouraged conversation, and offered reassurance when needed. It seemed to work out. Some patients were reassured, others would rather have been alone. No serious effects were observed. We could see no reasonable way out of this alteration in therapeutic technique covenant with therapeutic responsibility.

The monologues were another matter. They have no therapeutic justification. We wanted them and they have proved enlightening. Most patients hated them. Some sabotaged. The monologues were brief, mystifying to the patients, and, as nearly as we can see, a harmless annoyance. Something scientists do for their own reasons—like most laboratory tests.

The paper-and-pencil test was a break between the therapy and the return home. It interrupted the drug and the therapy and brought the patient back to reality. As such it probably interfered with some of the possible therapeutic effects of LSD but not with our psycholinguistic observations.

We were fortunate in our choice of attendants—graduate students in psychology of the same sex as the patient. They were generally sensitive and unintrusive. The sense the patients had of almost being hospitalized for a day allowed them to accept these people. In some cases, the attendants alleviated loneliness. Patients with families found them less welcome but never an embarrassment. They seemed to fit into the general rather awesome tone of the experiment and seemed to have no important consequence one way or another except insofar as they allowed us to use this drug on ambulatory patients outside of a hospital setting which would have destroyed the possibility of an LSD-facilitated analytic therapy entirely.

Appendix C

Release Form

Date ——

Dear Dr. Dahlberg:

You have suggested that it might be of value to my treatment if you were to administer the drug, lysergic acid diethylamide, to me in connection with my psychoanalysis. You have explained the nature of the drug to me and the reaction that it is capable of inducing, including the fact that it can produce certain transient physical side effects. In addition, you have explained to me the current status of the research reports regarding possible genetic damage from this drug and have offered me the opportunity to have my own chromosomal structure studied both before and after the course of LSD. You have encouraged me to consult with any lawyers, physicians, or other scientists before I undertake participating in this study. You have explained that the therapeutic use of lysergic acid diethylamide is a fairly recent development and that such use has had as yet neither extensive nor widespread application, and that you are offering me a chance to participate in a research project using lysergic acid diethylamide.

With full knowledge and understanding of all of the foregoing, I hereby consent to your use of lysergic acid diethylamide, and to the making and use for research purposes only of tape recordings in connections with my psychoanalysis, and in consideration of your making such use of the drug and recordings I hereby remise, release, and forever discharge you and your heirs, executors, and administrators from any and all causes or actions, claims, and damages whatsoever I or my heirs, executors, administrators, or personal representatives ever had, now have, or may hereafter have against you or them by reason of your use of lysergic acid diethylamide and recordings in connection with my psychoanalysis.

Witnessed: ———   *(Signature)*

Discussion by *Harold Kelman, M.D.*

My discussion reformulated as a proposition could read: good research is to good therapy as good therapy is to good research as both are to good investigation carried on by good people.

In 1912 Freud said, "It is indeed one of the distinctions of psychoanalysis that research and treatment proceed hand in hand, but still the technique required for the one begins at a certain point to diverge from that of the other."[1] I also believe that the longer that point of divergence is put off and the narrower the gap between the two remains, the better both will be.[2]

What can contribute to such possibilities? Briefly put, better people being better investigators using better techniques in their therapies and researches, being guided by better theories of man and better models for understanding and formulating the experimental setting we call the psychoanalytic situation.

Bridgman, who believed that creative science is essentially a "private rather than [a] public"[3] matter, hoped that someday we could invent an "introspectional microscope"[3] (p. 238) and the grammar to describe and organize what we saw. Using the phenomenological principle of the unbiased approach for observing, describing, and organizing the phenomena of internal states and external reality and unifying them through private creative science and public objective science, we could carry on clinical and experimental investigations. For doing so isolability of phenomena is prerequisite.

In Bridgman's terms, "Given an isolated enclosure and all the measurements that can be made inside of the enclosure as a function of time then these measurements will be found to be correlated into some sort of pattern"[3] (p. 188). The analytic situation is an isolated enclosure, functioning in time and following some sort of pattern, the internal and external constituents of which can be measured qualitatively in relative terms and quantitatively in numerical ones.

Some of Freud's other comments are pertinent here. He felt that "cases . . . destined at the start to scientific purposes and treated accordingly suffer in consequence; while the most successful cases are those in which one proceeds, as it were, aimlessly, and allows oneself to be overtaken by any surprises, always presenting to them an open mind, free from any expectations."[1] Although he mentioned the latter in connection with therapy, these attitudes apply equally to research and are inherent in the scientific attitude. It in turn is integral to the more effective use of the spectrum of methodologies appropriate to different stages of inquiry and varied according to the needs of the respective disciplines from astronomy to theology, from atomics to biology, to poetry.

A bit further on Freud adds, "The distinction here drawn between the two different attitudes would have no significance if we already possessed all the knowledge (or even the essential knowlededte) about the unconscious and the structure of the neuroses which is obtained by means of the analytic work."[1] Noteworthy is his reference to these attitudes as "mental" implying his definition of mental coming out of the "soft voice of the intellect," which was the tool by which knowledge was gained.

Our notion of knowledge in psychoanalysis has evolved since 1912. There is the accumulated body of knowledge we have gained since then. The philosophical premises of theory formulation have moved from rigid determinism applicable to closed systems based on a Newtonian mechanics to relative determinism operating in open systems hierarchically understood. From an insistence on strict causality we have moved to using acausal categories of operations and laws. From the individual as the sole variable in an otherwise static system dealing with ideal cases we now have methodologies for understanding the operations in and between two or more persons in moving fields influencing each other in flow patterns manifesting conditions of oscillating equilibrium. Briefly put, we now have holistic theories of human beings in moving fields in which system thinking can be applied and which take into account not only the individual but his extended environments, namely, the interpersonal and the intrapsychic reference as well.

Freud continued, "I cannot recommend my colleagues emphatically enough to take as a model in psycho-analytic treatment the surgeon who puts aside all his own feelings, including that of human sympathy, and concentrates his mind on one single purpose, that of performing the operation as skillfully as possible . . . . The justification for this coldness in feeling in the analyst is that it is the condition which brings the greatest advantage to both persons involved."[1] What happened in Freud exemplifies the impossibility of fulfilling his own admonition; other factors operating in him made it possible for him to recognise that impossibility and to make creative use of his observations of himself and others.

First came the requirement of personal analysis and later the suggestion for reanalysis every 5 yr. Then followed transference and subsequently countertransference. Also, in his actual therapeutic work Freud was hardly that paradigm of the cold surgeon, as has been amply documented in his relationship to the wolf-man[4] as but one of many such instances. The person of therapist as instrument kept demanding further investigation.

Discipline, rigor, precision, consistency, reliability, specification, and standardization, by himself and others, enhance the effectiveness of the investigator as researcher and therapist. They help him become more scientific and do not dehumanize him, in fact enhance his humaneness. I use "scientific" as understood not only in the natural but also in the life sciences and as defined by phenomenologists who give a nonphysicalistic interpretation of science.

In clinical medicine the standardization of the therapist's person has made great strides. In Feinstein's *Clinical Judgment* he demonstrates the clinician to be a "uniquely discriminating, adaptable, and portable scientific apparatus that can be calibrated" and who requires *self-standardization* of bedside performance to match . . . the assumed precision of non-clinical colleagues."[5] Kanzer and Blum suggest that in psychoanalysis "the era of scientific validation is drawing closer"[6] with the recognition of "the need to standardize the analyst himself as a judge of analyzability"[6] (p. 135). They suggest that with these might come "the standardization of the training of that ultimate instrument of psychoanalytic therapy, the analyst himself"[6] (p. 140), an objective also shadowed by the dangers of dogma and dehumanization.

Using the phenomenological approach I feel that those legitimate concerns that are confronted and forms of standardization that are used which derive from the analyst's humanness increase his humaneness and not only his effectiveness but possibly also his wisdom. I can only list here the seven attitudes and nine modes of being I have developed elsewhere which, when aspired to as ultimates, will maximize his effectiveness as investigator of himself and others while carrying on investigation as therapy and research.[7] Six of these attitudes I have taken from Martin, modified them and added a seventh. They are the nonteleological attitude, unconventionality, unobtrusiveness, incorruptibility, being respectfully vigilant, threshold conscious, and choiceless aware.

The nine modes of being are described in the form of paradoxes which have been used since man's search for information, knowledge, and wisdom began. They are passionate objectivity concomitant with dispassionate subjectivity; simultaneously moving toward the ultimate of the personal and the impersonal, which are equivaalents of each other; being open to action in nonaction concomitant with nonaction in action; being moved by the will power of desirelessness; being moved by moral toughness and moral compassion integral to each other and to moral courage; being open to experiencing tension producing and reducing as natural oscillations and to conflicting and cooperating systems operating in hierarchies; being simultaneously at his own core as well as that of the other; and all the time being responsive to and containing dualistic and nondualistic theories and techniques.

As the person of the investigator, as therapist, researcher, and instrument, moves toward the foregoing ultimates, he will also experience and use techniques, in his investigations, from the ultimate of pure technique with reference to the ultimate of objectification of an aspect of the system of the whole as pure object and ideal case, to being an expression of techniqueless moments in therapy as kairos[8] and in research as creative intuition.[9] This spectrum of categories of technique is the outcome of my detailed phenomenologic response to the question "what is technique?"[2]

I feel what I have defined with reference to the person of the investigator, as therapist and researcher, the psychoanalytic situation, the models he uses, the techniques he applies, and the theories of man that guide him makes it possible to longer delay the point of divergence of therapy and research and to keep the gap between the two narrower than was possible in 1912.

In the instance of investigation cited by Dr. Dahlberg and Jaffe I find that they have moved implicitly and explicitly in the directions I have defined and that they have in a measure affirmed my original proposition. I find them to be good people doing good investigation in which the focus on research did not proceed at the expense of good therapy.

References

1. Freud, S.: Recommendations for physicians on the psycho-analytic method of treatment (1912). In: Collected Papers, Vol. II. London, Hogarth Press, 1933, pp. 326, 327.
2. Kelman, H.: What is technique? In: Helping People: Karen Horney's Psychoanalytic Approach. New York, Science House, 1971, Chap. 28.
3. Bridgman, P. W.: The Way Things Are. New York, The Viking Press, 1961, Chap. 92, p. V.
4. Gardiner, W.: The Wolf-Man. New York, Basic Books, 1970.
5. Feinstein, A. R.: Clinical Judgment. Baltimore, William & Wilkins, 1967. Review in J.A.M.A. 201:985, 1967.
6. Kanzer, M., and Blum, H. P.: Clinical psychoanalysis since 1939. In: Wolman, B. B. (Ed.): Psychoanalytic Techniques. New York, Basic Books, 1967, p. 133.
7. Cf. reference 2, Chap. 9.
8. Kelman, H.: "Kairos" and the therapeutic process. J. Exist. 1: (Summer) 1960; "Kairos": The auspicious moment. Amer. J. Psychoanal. 19:59–83, 1969; Helping People. New York, Science House, 1971, Chaps. 27 and 28.
9. Kelman, H.: Creative talent and creative passion in therapy. Amer. J. Psychoanal. 23:133–141, 1963.

East Meets West: Moritist and Freudian Psychotherapies

DAVID REYNOLDS, PH.D.

JOE YAMAMOTO, M.D.

In the early twentieth century two creative personalities on opposite sides of the globe made, independently, efforts to break away from neurological explanations of neurosis. These men had much in common: they personally experienced mental anguish, worked through their own cures, and developed strong, free characters. They learned to *listen* to the verbalizations of their patients and evolved models of the mind, psychic suffering, and cure based on their own experiences and their patients' descriptions of their experiences. There gathered around them a group of followers among whom special areas of interest were carved out for advanced exploration and expertise. There developed "schools" and "neo"-orthodoxies and a constant effort to make understandable the founders' basic contributions to the understanding of man amid changing social definitions of "reality."

Although the name of Sigmund Freud is familiar to us all, how many of you are aware of the name of the Japanese professor of psychiatry Morita Shōma, whom this brief sketch fits equally well?

The perceptions of man and neurosis underlying these two men's theoretical and practical concerns reflect well the sociocultural milieu in which they were formulated.

187

Freud's methods fit well within the Western traditions valuing rational-ity, individual expressiveness, and self-dependence or independence. In a broad sense, it can be said that Freud taught us that man can control his neurotic symptoms by understanding them in depth and detail, by expressing emotions in proper ways, and by weaning himself from un-productive relationships and the survivals of past unproductive relationships.

On the other hand, Morita's theory and method were conceived in an Eastern and, particularly, a Zen Buddhist tradition. They well reflect the Buddhist-related concerns of naturalistic acceptance of phenomenological reality, controlled attention, intuitive-experiential knowledge, social productivity, and familistic sharing.

Perhaps at this point it would be useful to outline the Moritist under-standing of neurosis and cure and to describe some of the methods that are employed today by Morita therapists in Japan.

Moritist writings abound with illustrations relating theory simply to our own experience. One such illustration may be useful here. Many of us have experienced the inner debate between getting up from beneath warm covers on a cold wintry day or remaining a bit longer in the warmth. As we lie debating, our day's work and play remain undone. This inner conflict resulting in unproductive inactivity is the essence of neurosis. Its roots lie in the misdirection of our attention away from the immediate tasks that, in a sense, "pull" us to complete them. Our attention is refocused on the inner struggle, on the avoidance of the momentary discomfort involved in getting up, on the effort to make ourselves "want" to get up. Thus, to some degree, we are all somewhat neurotic. Change the circum-stances slightly—a boy confronts a girl and flees from shyness, a woman refuses to leave her bed for fear she has cancer, a teacher cannot face his class nor a speaker his audience, a young man cannot work at his office for fear his boss will be displeased with his output—these are some of the forms of neurosis that a Moritist may deal with. In each case the patient's attention has been misdirected from the task at hand and refocused inward. Such is the nature of all neurosis, according to Moritist theory.

One might say that the neurotic person is "experientially unrealistic." He wants to resolve problems without facing them, he wants to find inner solutions where direct activity is the only reasonable course open to him, he desires perfection from an imperfect being in an imperfect world, and, finally, he seems not to be aware that other humans face similar imper-fections daily without being distracted by them.

We have no time to discuss the biological and behavioral sources of this misfocused-attention kernel of neurosis or the elaborations of diminished self-esteem, interpersonal difficulties, and progressive withdrawal that usually accompany it. Suffice it to say that the patient who presents himself for inpatient treatment at a Moritist hospital is likely to be shy, introverted, socially withdrawn, unhappy, and unproductive.

After the necessary business of admission is carried out, the typical patient begins the first phase of treatment. He is required to lie on a *futon* (Japanese mattress and quilt bedding) in a room by himself for 1 wk. During this period he is not allowed to converse, to smoke, to read, to write, to listen to the radio, or to engage in any other sort of recreational activity. He is permitted to take three meals a day, bathe once during the week, and take care of other natural and hygienic functions such as going to the bathroom, washing his face (once a day), and brushing his teeth. The senior author underwent a full week of absolute bed rest as part of his experiential approach to research.

One of the primary functions of this "absolute bed rest period" is to force the patient to encounter *himself* with minimal distraction. He must face himself with all his shortcomings, anxieties, and ruminations. He is instructed to accept whatever feelings and thoughts bubble to the surface of awareness. He learns experientially that waves of emotion come and go, thoughts follow one another without conscious control, appearing from nothing and disappearing into nothing.

A second function is to teach the patient experientially that the withdrawal from social interaction and activity (which seemed so desirable and "safe" when he entered the week of bed rest) is really an unnatural and uncomfortable experience. The boredom mounts during the last few days of bed rest so that when one is handed a broom and instructed to sweep out the room it is with a feeling of wholehearted joy that the task is undertaken. A kind of rebirth is reflected in the freshness of sensory experience, the sheer pleasure of moving about.

Thus, the second phase of treatment begins. The patient is assigned light manual tasks and is encouraged to find other tasks with which to occupy himself. He is to direct his attention to getting the job done. He is warned that the joy will pass, too, that feelings are changeable "like the Japanese sky." Life is not to be based on *feelings* but on productive activity. One can build a sense of self-worth on what he has accomplished—especially what he has accomplished for others.

Again, time prevents us from describing in detail more aspects of treatment. For example, the patient writes a diary each evening in which the doctor makes written comments during the day. There are group meetings and outings and various forms of posthospitalization contact. The entire course of therapy is carried out within a more-or-less familistic milieu.

With this descriptive background, we now turn to some interesting parallels between Freud's and Morita's conceptions of neurosis. It may be that by finding such common features in psychotherapies of various cultures we can begin to build on a "metalevel" a truly intercultural theory of neurosis and cure.

First, it seems clear that both theorists were building models of neurosis founded on the misdirection of psychic interest. They diverged somewhat in their specifications of the nature of the misdirection. For Freud it was tied to the service of repression. For Morita it was tied up in a sort of obsession with the self.

In both cases, then, cure is to be achieved by releasing this misdirected interest. Each individual is assumed to be capable of changing and therefore coping more appropriately. In both cases, this redirection is brought about in part at least by inner adjustments, often attitudinal adjustments. Self-acceptance is sought, be it acceptance of a self with lustful ideas and impulses or acceptance of a self with anxieties and imperfections. Relations with others may be reinterpreted to permit greater flexibility and spontaneity of behavior (though the limits of spontaneity are quite differently defined in the United States and Japan).

On the other hand, there are some critical contrasts that may be drawn between the two systems. There are conditions under which increased self-knowledge is to be avoided in Morita therapy. For example, group discussion of symptoms may promote self-knowledge at the risk of focusing more attention on the self and inhibiting cure.

An ever clearer divergence is apparent in the two systems' definitions of cure. Freudians tend to see cure in terms of being symptom free, i.e., feeling better. Moritists tend to see cure in terms of being socially productive. That is, a patient can leave a Moritist hospital with fears and anxieties and obsessions similar to those with which he entered, yet be considered by all concerned "cured." If he is able to function in the midst of his misery he is well. And he may consider himself a better man than those of us who function without the limitations that "reality" has imposed upon him. And it may well be that when reality imposes the 'imitations of injury, old age, loss of loved ones, loss of a successful clinical practice, impending death, or whatever, such a man is better equipped than we are to cope with life within the new boundaries.

One final difference worth mentioning but difficult to communicate lies in the kinds of self-knowledge that the two systems emphasize. It is our impression that Freudian psychotherapies stress more rational and interpretable symbolic forms of knowledge—such knowledge can usually be transmitted verbally. On the other hand, Moritist psychotherapies stress intuitive, essentially nonrational understandings that are best realized experientially through behavior. We recognize that both systems use both approaches to self-knowledge but the difference in emphasis seems important.

Much can be said about the relative advantages and disadvantages of insight-oriented versus acceptance-oriented psychotherapies. Depending on the patient's problems and capacities, insight therapy may be impractical or even harmful. On the other hand, acceptance at a low level of functioning may be second best to dealing with the *sources* of unhappiness once they are made known.

At any rate psychotherapies are creations of their social milieu as well as their founder. And, at least in the Western world, they survive in a social milieu that they in turn have helped to create. In a Japan increasingly influenced by Western ideas of the nature of man and society, well-being and discomfort, Moritist principles are being reinterpreted to fit the changing understandings of therapies and patients. It will be interesting to see if and how Western psychotherapies can profit from increased familiarity with Eastern ways of thought.

Discussion

Two physicians have advocated quite different treatment approaches for neurotic patients. Both used the powerful motivation of the neurotic sufferer to improve. Freud used an outpatient approach and utilized the power of the transference to foster self-understanding as the goal. Morita devised an inpatient treatment approach without great emphasis on theoretical bases for his approach. His goal was more functionally and pragmatically oriented toward regaining the ability to work. Such a goal is valued in itself in Japan with the cultural emphasis on the importance of contributing to the family, group, and nation. The specific methods used are based upon Zen Buddhism and also perhaps European medical traditions with the authority of the physician-healer. These techniques seem to have been tailored for the needs of some neurotic patients in Japan.

The senior author actually experienced the initial bed rest phase of treatment. He did not feel frustrated or as unhappy as the therapists explained that he might; however, he did find himself anticipating and finding pleasure in such ordinarily routine activities as going to the bathroom or being permitted to brush his teeth and wash his face!

The junior author, inexperienced in the Morita therapy situation, asked himself, how would I feel in the hospital? Here, the answer was closer to the detailed explanation of the Morita therapist. The Japanese grow up in personal contact with their mothers. Until beginning school, each child is within eyesight of and solicitous contact with the mother. This being the case, separation is not ordinarily experienced by the Japanese child. The child sleeps in the same room with the family on beds made on the floor. There is much affectionate contact with the child. Both father and mother believe that the child's needs are important and make efforts to see that the child is happy and growing. He becomes aware of his status in the family.

Of course, as he grows older, the child is taught the limits of acceptable behavior and the importance of his obligations and responsibilities. He is told to behave in a manner reflecting credit on his parents and clan. Acceptable actions are necessary to avoid being laughed at or being confronted with social disapproval. Such disapproval can be directed not only against oneself, but also against one's family and clan. The child is told, "You must behave or they will all laugh at you." Consider how close this is to the patient's neurotic fears!

Morita therapy, with the initial phase of social isolation, a condition quite alien to most Japanese, then utilizes the motivating force of a stressful situation. To be alone means not to be aware of all the social cues learned through a lifetime to maintain social grace. To be alone means to be a stranger in one's own land.

Perhaps you can see that the first phase of bed rest can be worse than the prison on one's own neurosis. You might ask then, why doesn't the patient leave? Most Japanese patients have learned to *gamman* (to be patient and to persevere). There is also the factor of face, that one does not drop out!

Given this hellish first phase, the *sensei* (learned teacher) comes to the rescue. He has the answer. He knows the way back to social grace. He conducts group discussions in which the new attitude of acceptance of one's symptoms is taught. The patient becomes able to cope with his anxieties for he learns to work. In the process, he feels worthwhile and becomes again a part of a family, the Morita hospital family. There are gains in self-esteem and in social acceptance. The patient may be neurotic, but he learns that in this family, it does not matter as long as he can work and relate to his family. In recognizing the value of this new way of life, he becomes an active member of a large new family with reinforcement of enthusiastic acceptance of a new sense of group identity.

Discussion by Norman J. Levy, M.D.

At a time when many people still stress differences between the East and West, Drs. Reynolds and Yamamoto have tried to share with us a more balanced picture, indicating similarities as well as differences. For example, they point out the traditional differences which have led Dr. Akihisa Kondo,[1] who is presenting a paper at almost this very time in Tokyo on *Several Characteristics of Morita Therapy in Comparison with Psychoanalytic-Psychotherapy,* to observe that the closeness and similarity of Morita's ideas with the Japanese culturally inherited ideas make his therapy "more easily understood and accepted with more intimacy by the patients than perhaps by the Western oriented medical people."

The authors state that Freudian psychotherapists stress more rational and interpretable symbol forms of knowledge whereas Moritists focus more on the intuitive, essentially nonrational understandings that are best realized experientially. Kondo, who studied with Horney at the American Institute for Psychoanalysis and who has been in continuous communication with Kelman at the Postgraduate Center for Mental Health, states that the Morita therapist believes that "man is bestowed with a life force by which he can develop himself," that he is "inherently oriented for self actualization," and that "living in and with the flow of the life force does not only mean a spontaneous creative way of life," but also living it "without dissecting it by the static pattern of subjects against objects." Man is caught in conflict between his subjective egocentric drives and the objective reality of life. This conflict leads to the attempt to make the impossible possible. The attempt impoverishes life because it restricts man's possibility of experiencing the wholeness of the processes of living. He is opposed to thinking in terms of dichotomies such as either/or and prefers terms of both/and. Morita claimed that Freud's libido theory was too speculative, partial, and dubious. For him the life force was analogous to Horney's[2] concept of the real self, "that central inner force, common to all human beings and yet unique in each which is the deep source of growth." Kondo points out that in making the unconscious conscious the Freudians stress the notion that knowledge reached by the process of free association leads to transformation. This knowledge is arrived at through detecting and exposing the pathology of the patient and bringing it to his attention in order to help him acquire insight. Kondo holds that the Freudian therapist is out to exorcise and eradicate the pathological part so that health will be restored. In contrast, Morita was critical of the split of the subject into subject and object through self-reflection because, for him, when the self was not self-conscious, it was healthy. Morita believed that the mobilizing of the spontaneous life force could never be achieved by intellectual understanding or persuasion in an analyst's office; it must be directly achieved by actual living in a limited situation. His concern was "centered on how to help the patient accomplish self liberation and live fully here and now." Morita was not so much interested in having the patient involved in finding out traumatic experiences or other causes in the past regarding his sickness. He desired to prepare the patient to experience his spontaneous desire for activity, thus enchancing his participation in the external world, natural and human. He did not deny the value of verbal communication but stressed the importance of understanding by direct emotional experiences. These experiences enabled the patient to develop a more realistic and spontaneous attitude toward life. This direct contact with the actual reality in activity by jumping into it and experiencing the mental and emotional processes in the stream of life had for him a greater therapeutic effect than dealing with verbal images in an office.

When the authors state Morita's goal was "more functionally and pragmatically oriented toward regaining the ability to work," I believe they are oversimplifying the aims of Morita therapy. As Kumasaka[3] put it, in Morita therapy the therapist is "nature," the psychiatrist is only a teacher who assists the patient in gaining insight into his position in nature. He indicates that cultural differences between East and West impose a serious obstacle for communicating about Morita therapy. In the East nature is to be accepted "as it is," whereas in the West nature is something to be challenged and conquered. In the West, to accept it is to be considered a defeatist. Both Kondo and I[4] believe that certain concepts of Morita therapy can be reframed according to psychoanalytic concepts and be useful adjuncts to psychoanalytic procedure, especially with those patients who are under the tyranny of the shoulds and are compulsively driven to use living in the imagination, supremacy of the mind, and alienation from feelings as solutions to conflict.

The authors speak of Freudians seeing cure in terms of being symptom free, whereas the Moritists see it in terms of being socially productive. Speaking as one who subscribes to the views of Horney, Kelman, and those of similar persuasion, I wish to present Horney's[5] position that the word cure is appropriate only as long as we think of relief of a symptom like a phobia or an insomnia. But we cannot "cure" the wrong course which the development of a person has taken. We can only assist him in gradually outgrowing his difficulties so that his development may assume a more constructive course. We can talk in terms of aims and goals. Those of Morita therapy are for the more immediate present, those of psychoanalysis for the long range of deeper characterological change.

The authors indicate that the aims of both are to enable man to find himself and his place in society. They correctly state that the customary limits of flexibility and spontaneity are quire differently defined in Japan and in the West. In Japan, however, there has been increasing interest not only in Freud, Adler, and Jung, but also in Fromm, Horney, Kelman, Menninger, Rogers, Sullivan, and their colleagues. Just as Western attitudes and concepts about psychoanalysis are not static, so the thoughts and techniques of Morita's followers are evolving. I believe that, with the increasing influence of Western thought in Japan, the limits of spontaneity will more closely approximate each other, at least among some of the more progressive groups. Current Western interest in brief psychotherapy, encounter groups, and primal therapy with the focus on new techniques to achieve more speedy contact with deep feelings makes me wonder whether, in the near future, someone in the West might not try to apply the principles of Morita therapy with a group of his patients. How effective such a technique would be is open to question. In 1959 Kelman[6] wondered about the authoritarian aspects of the treatment. Iwai and Reynolds,[7] however, wrote that, in any country, relatively strong authority can be accepted if both interactors feel it is in the best interest of the subordinate member.

Kelman, in "Communing and Relating,"[8] "Oriental Psychological Processes,"[9] and other articles in the *American Journal of Psychoanalysis* and in his new book, *Helping People*,[10] contends that "many aspects of Eastern wisdom are not alien to the West and that many occidentals are now more open and available to what the East has to offer." He specifically discusses ways in which Western psychotherapies can profit from increased familiarity with Eastern ways of thought. In fact, he states that ultimately psychoanalysis is more Eastern in its technique, aims, and aspirations than Western. He notes that it is not Eastern in its theories, however, but that psycho-analysis and its theories are a product of the West, of the subject-object dualism in thought, and that between theory and technique there is a built-in dichotomy. In his work on communing and relating, phenomenology, existentialism, and utilization of Eastern ways of approach to resolving neurotic processes, Kelman has been trying to expand increasingly the experiential aspects of the therapeutic process.

Last, the authors refer to the doctor as one who has the answers and guides the patient back to social grace. Kondo,[11] in writing about the doctor-patient relationship in Morita therapy, states that therapists who obtain the most effective clinical results are those who have themselves suffered from this kind of neurosis and who have had the experience of outgrowing and overcoming it. As a result they have a genuine, accepting, sympathetic attitude toward the patient. They can understand and accept him and are in the best position to enable him to develop self-acceptance and a realistic attitude toward life. This is somewhat different from the concept proposed by Freud of the therapist being impenetrable to the patient, like a mirror, reflecting nothing but what is shown to him. It is more in the spirit of Kelman,[10] who wrote in 1955 that the therapeutic situation is a bipolar unitary process, a constant and continuous, mutually and reciprocally influencing human situation since doctor and patient are in and of the environment of each other.

References

1. Kondo, A.: Morita's Shinkeishitsu and His Therapy. Tokyo, 1971. To be published.
2. Horney, K.: Neurosis and Human Growth. New York, W. W. Norton, 1950, p. 17.
3. Kumasaka, Y.: Discussion of Kora, T.: Morita therapy. Int. J. Psychiat. 1:641–642, 1965.
4. Levy, N.: Discussion of Kora, T.: Morita therapy. Int. J. Psychiat. 1:642–643, 1965.
5. Horney, K.: *Op. cit.,* p. 333.
6. Kelman, H.: Psychotherapy in the Far East. In: Masserman, J., and Moreno, J. L. (Eds.): Social Psychotherapy, Vol. IV of Progress in Psychotherapy. New York, Grune & Stratton, 1959, pp. 296–313.
7. Iwai, H., and Reynolds, D.: Morita psychotherapy: The views from the West. Amer. J. Psychiat. 126:155–160, 1970.
8. Kelman, H.: Communing and relating. Amer. J. Psychoanal. 18:77–98, 158–170, 1958; 19:73–105, 188–215, 1959.
9. Kelman, H.: Oriental psychological processes. Amer. J. Psychoanal. 23:67–84, 1963.
10. Kelman, H.: Helping People. New York, Science House, 1971.
11. Kondo, A.: The doctor-patient relationship in Morita therapy. Jap. J. Psycho-anal. 7:6, 1961.
12. Kelman, H.: The doctor-patient relationship in therapy. Amer. J. Psychoanal. 15:16–19, 1955.

The Technology of Psychotherapy*

HANS H. STRUPP, PH.D.

In this chapter I propose to explore certain basic conditions surrounding an individual's lasting psychological influence on another. In psychotherapy (under which I continue to subsume psychoanalysis as a major subform) the resulting personality and behavior changes are ordinarily described as "therapeutic"; however, it will be seen that the approach has broad implications for child rearing, education, rehabilitation, correction—in short, for any area which is concerned with the promotion of personality growth, the development of mature, self-directing, autonomous, and responsible adults who under ordinary circumstances can conduct their own affairs and are not in need of help, support, or guidance from others or society at large. As a corollary, I believe that the exploration of this psychological influence is the basic task facing the researcher in psychotherapy, to which the study of techniques per se is secondary. Conceptual clarification of these issues is an essential prerequisite for further meaningful research in this area.

*Reprinted from Archives of General Psychiatry 26:220–228, 1972, with the permission of author and publisher, and exceptional acceptance by the American Academy of Psychoanalysis.

Background

On the basis of my previous research efforts in psychotherapy I recently outlined a two-pronged attack on exploring the nature of the psychotherapeutic
influence. On the one hand, I addressed myself to the problem of *what*
is learned by the patient in psychotherapy, concluding that therapeutic
learning proceeds on a broad front and that in all forms of psychotherapy
a variety of things are learned by the patient, ranging from the overcoming
of anxieties to the acquisition of greater self-control, new strategies of
dealing with interpersonal events, and so on.[1] On the other hand, I dealt
further with the nature of the psychotherapist's influence and the conditions
that must be created for therapeutic learning to occur.[2] In the latter paper
I drew attention to the importance of the therapist's *control* over the patient
and his interpersonal behavior, elaborating to some extent on the conditions I consider necessary for therapeutic learning to occur. In this connection, I also dealt with the distinction between "specific" (technique) and
"nonspecific" (broad interpersonal) factors, arguing that their relative
importance has never been adequately tested, and allowing for the strong
possibility (stressed by Frank[3] and Shapiro[4]) that the weight of the therapeutic influence is carried by the latter factors, often referred to as "placebo
effects." Whatever the contribution of so-called nonspecific factors to
psychotherapeutic change may be, it is essential to make the ingredients
increasingly explicit. In the recent past I have become interested in the
problem of suggestibility (and its counterpart suggestion or suggestiveness),
a concept I consider as obscure as placebo effects or nonspecific factors.
On closer inspection it may turn out that these concepts are in fact closely
related, and that they account in large part for the essential ingredients
of what is ordinarily called the psychotherapeutic process. Again we are
faced with the basic questions: (a) What factors in the patient make him
susceptible to the influence of the psychotherapist (influencer, healer,
physician, parent, etc.); and (b) what factors at the disposal of the psychotherapist enable him to exert an effect on the patient's suggestibility,
persuasibility, amenability to social influence? Phrasing the questions
in this way carries no implication that any forthcoming explanation will
clarify everything about the psychotherapeutic enterprise—Kenneth Mark
Colby cogently observed that no "all" exists about anything—but I submit
that clarification of these problems will go a long way toward unraveling
the mystery still surrounding the nature of the psychotherapeutic influence
and the problem of therapeutic change. In the ensuing discussion I shall
make a renewed attempt to come to grips with the problem.

Freud's disservice: A historical note

Certain terms in the area of psychotherapy have acquired the connotation of "dirty" words, with the result that the phenomena to which they refer have ceased to be respectable; furthermore, and more serious, such value judgments have had the effect of delaying or even deterring exploration. Prominent among these terms, for present purposes, are: placebo effect and suggestion. The blame for denigrating the concepts of suggestion and suggestibility must be placed at Freud's doorstep.

Freud's early interest in hypnosis and the evolution of psychoanalysis as a set of therapeutic techniques hardly bears repetition. It is important to point out, however, that as Freud came to develop his basic concepts and the model of the psychoanalytic situation, he proceeded to draw a sharp distinction between psychoanalysis and other treatment approaches which, in his judgment, were "merely" based on suggestion. The neurotic patient's tendency to transfer infantile patterns of behavior, expectations, and fantasies to the therapist was seen as part and parcel of his "suggestibility," and indeed the core of his "illness." (I shall return to this formulation later.) Psychoanalysis was designed, through dissection and neutralization of the patient's resistances, to deprive him of this "weapon." In his later writings Freud admitted that the therapist does use suggestion but insisted that the thrust of the analytic technique was focused upon persuading the patient to relinquish his resistances by demonstrating to him that they were mal-adaptive and rooted in infantile experiences, fantasies, and misconceptions, hence anachronistic and unnecessary. Thus, the therapist supposedly did not "manipulate" (another "dirty" word)* the transference relationship but he analyzed it. The model Freud was inveighing against, I believe, was that of the domineering hypnotist who was bombarding the patient with authoritarian commands, and he was (very commendably) advocating a permissive situation in which, ideally, the patient is encouraged to seek and find his own answers. Whatever the merits of Freud's distinction, the fact remains that the therapist exerts a powerful psychological influence on the patient, and it appears that the analytic situation was precisely designed to augment, intensify, and potentiate it. In fact, by creating a paradoxical situation in therapy which is ostensibly a relationship between

---

*Since the main thrust of this paper will predictably be criticized on these grounds, it is important to stress the dictionary definition of the word manipulate: "to handle, manage or use, especially with skill, in some process of treatment or performance." I submit that this is precisely what psychotherapy is and what the patient has a right to expect.

two adults but which is also conducive to stimulating the reemergence of infantile patterns, Freud forged an exceedingly powerful tool for personality and behavior change.

Freud's distinction had of course the strategic advantage of extolling the uniqueness of psychoanalytic psychotherapy over all contenders, notably the crude practices which must have been extant at the time. In the long run, psychoanalysts could feel comfortably secure in the belief that they were practicing a superior brand of psychotherapy and that the psychological mechanisms they utilized in the patient or brought to bear on the interaction were qualitatively different from anyone else's. This belief, in case anyone doubts, is still widespread and neatly serves to undergird the analyst's professional grandiosity and presumption. The latter was scarcely Freud's intention, but his formulations had the effect of sequestering the psychotherapeutic influence as something "special" in human relations, thereby inhibiting inquiries designed to investigate what it might have *in common* with other techniques of psychological influence. Only in relatively recent years have attempts been made to bring about "translations" (e.g., Alexander,[5] Dollard and Miller[6]).

The patient's susceptibility to psychological influence

What are the factors in the patient (pupil, delinquent, medical patient, normal person) that render him susceptible to psychological influence or, alternatively, vitiate a therapist's efforts? I view this susceptibility as a universal continuum ranging from high susceptibility to virtual insusceptibility.

Childhood antecedents. It is quite likely that part of the susceptibility to social influence is biologically determined, that is, "wired" into the human organism, but in any case it is a basic tendency present soon after birth and of course heavily reinforced by mothering behavior in infancy and early childhood. As a result of early experiences the human infant under ordinary circumstances becomes highly susceptible and responsive to social cues, particularly if, we must surmise, the experience is perceived as intrinsically gratifying. Thus the child becomes dependent upon and seeks to perpetuate social interactions which are conducive to his receiving love, approval, and other rewards. He develops "basic trust," which also embodies blind faith in, and obedience to, a powerful external (parental) authority. Freud was undoubtedly correct in asserting that the adult's faith in God is a derivative of the child's sense of fear, awe, unquestioned submission, obedience, and helplessness vis-à-vis an all-powerful

parent figure. In turn, these feelings may be rooted in the child's own narcissistic fantasies of omnipotence. Throughout life the human being strives for
independence and emancipation from these feelings while at the same time
(because of his inherent weakness, finiteness, and fear of death) remaining
forever vulnerable to reversion. It is this basic substrate upon which any
influencer—therapist, physician, judge, educator, priest, leader, expert,
or society at large—capitalizes by placing himself, often only temporarily,
in the position of an all-powerful authority who exercises more or less
complete control over the subject. More accurately, he encourages (manipulates) the subject to accept him in that position from which he then proceeds
to exert his influence. It is clear that whenever the subject is ill, weak, help-
less, or feels dependent (for many reasons) or ignorant (as all of us are in a
multitude of areas), the stage is set for persons or organizations in authority
to influence him. The psychoanalytic concept of regression refers to the same
phenomenon. It is also clear, to cite but one example, that a patient in a
state of crisis is highly amenable to the therapist's interventions (i.e., he is
highly "motivated" to be influenced) and that such situations are typically
coupled with the arousal of (primitive) affect.*

In short, under ordinary circumstances a child acquires a basic
personality trait of suggestibility, persuasibility, educability, and psychological modifiability (treatability, "analyzability") in later life. Hypno-
tizability is probably part of this constellation. Once acquired, this tendency
is exceedingly stable and persistent. Further, the strong human desire
to belong to a group, to conform to its morals and mores, and to be approved
and loved by persons in authority (and one's peers) appears to be an integral
part of the susceptibility to social influence.† It is clear that the psychotherapeutic enterprise, not to mention education, religion, and propaganda, among others, is squarely built upon the supposition that most
people are susceptible to, and influenceable by, psychological means, that
they change attitudes, behavior, beliefs, etc., as a response to such techniques provided certain conditions are met. At the same time, however,
people are more or less "resistant" to such influences.

Part of the reason for this resistance is the development of a "self-
system," "ego," or whatever terminology may be employed to characterize

*It has recently been pointed out that the contemporary phenomenon of the "Jesus
revolution" among alienated youth represents another version of the search for a
benevolent paternal authority which many of the followers have never experienced.
    †Highly pertinent to this discussion seems to be the finding reported by Josephine
Hilgard[7] that good hypnotic subjects appear to have a family background characterized
in part by strict discipline in the context of a warm, loving parent-child relationship.

the emergence a person's self-directing, executive tendencies and his striving for autonomy and independence. It suffices to note that many impulses, wishes, strivings, etc., are gradually brought under self-control, concomitant the erosion or diminution of parental control. Nevertheless, the susceptibility to social cues remains present and perenially latent in everyone. Indeed, social living would be impossible without it.

Defense mechanisms, resistance and transference tendencies

1. *The "normal solution."* There is reason to believe that when early experiences have been essentially satisfying, the growing child will partly assimilate ("introject") the control exerted by his parents and build his own control mechanisms; partly he will remain open and, under appropriate conditions, receptive to similar kinds of social influence; partly he will reject and become resistant to attempts by others to control him. Thus, the "normal" child will become educable, teachable, adaptable, and, within limits, influenceable. At the same time, the acquisition of self-control must be seen as a major milestone in human development; it is largely a matter of how the growing human being responds to external constraints (discipline) and how he learns to discipline himself.* The implications of the "normal solution" will emerge more clearly in the light of two broad classes of abortive attempts.

2. *The "neurotic solution."* The individual becomes "neurotic"; that is, for complex reasons which have been amply discussed in the literature, he declares war on the mediators of social influence (usually his parents) and by means of various autonomic (unconscious) strategies and tactics seeks to ward off their influence by controlling them. He fights against submission, obedience, conformity, and compliance while at the same time craving them for the purpose of winning the parents' love and approval. In short, he becomes "conflicted."

3. *The "psychopathic solution."* The individual largely rejects the parental influence without first having assimilated the morals and values of the cultural group the parents represent. Such individuals do not grow out of the confines of the parental influence after having submitted to it in a deep sense; instead they reject it or pay only superficial allegiance to it. This group of individuals is exemplified by psychopaths and other "rebels." Traditionally, they have been considered very unpromising patients for

---

Waelder[8] epitomized the dilemma of child rearing in these terms: how to love without spoiling and how to discipline without traumatizing.

psychotherapy, which makes good sense if the therapeutic relationship presupposes at least a rudimentary willingness on the patient's part to relive some parts—usually painful parts—of his childhood. These people are frequently described as having poor "impulse control," being given to antisocial "acting out," flaunting accepted moral standards, and preferring immediate gratification to what the adequately socialized person has come to accept as delays in gratification, and they are considered insensitive to the feelings of others.

To sum it up, the normal individual has "come to terms" with the problem of social influence and has succeeded in modulating it; the neurotic continues to make an issue of it; and the psychopath has largely turned his back on it. With regard to later attempts at social influence, it would follow that the neurotic person is the most vulnerable of the three types precisely for the reason that he remains entangled in the issue of whether in interpersonal relationships he will fight for his independence (which often turns out to be a pseudoindependence) or whether he will abjectly submit to a feared authority figure (couched by Freud in terms of homosexual surrender and "passivity").

The feat of therapeutic penetrance

The concept of "basic trust" may be seen as referring to the child's pristine and uncritical openness to social influence, his primitive yet pervasive faith in the goodness and beneficence of the nurturing adults, and his willingness to surrender to their unlimited power. This attitude is profoundly illustrated by Jesus' last words: "Father, into thy hands I commit my spirit" [Luke 23:46]. To anticipate my thesis, I will argue that the crucial context for significant therapeutic change lies precisely in a semblance of this attitude which is concomitant with the (however temporary) complete abandonment of so-called defense mechanisms in relation to a healer experienced as possessing superior powers. Such complete submission, however, is extremely painful and occurs only under great duress. Furthermore, it is undergone only if it promises to liberate the individual from isolation by letting him become a full-fledged adult. The full implications of this observation need to be explored further.

Conversely, traditional defense mechanisms may be viewed as more or less adaptive techniques to regulate the extent to which the person will be susceptible to psychological influence from powerful authority figures. They may also be seen as mechanisms for controlling oneself and others. In this light, the psychoanalytic emphasis on analyzing the patient's defenses makes good sense: By gradually eroding his habitual ("characterological") techniques for fighting off another person's influence by controlling him, the therapist "opens up" the patient and, typically against the patient's "will," paves the way for personality and behavior change. Time and again he forces the patient to experience the inutility and self-defeating character of his resistive maneuvers and, paradoxically, coerces him into renewed experiences of basic trust.

How does the therapist accomplish the feat of eroding the patient's defenses against being influenced by a powerful parent figure? The following appear to be basic components of the overall strategy:

1. The patient turns to the therapist for help. He is driven by suffering and unhappiness to accept the advice, counsel, and ministrations of a healer-expert. If he is deeply distressed and propelled by inner forces (not by relatives, a court of law, etc.) to seek help from another person, he tends to be "motivated" to subordinate himself to a healer. On a deeper level, because of early childhood experiences, he seeks to reinstitute a parent-child situation in which he is taken care of, loved, forgiven, encouraged, coaxed, and so on. It may be hypothesized that the greater the reservoir of happy, rewarding experiences in early childhood—no matter how much they may be obscure or overlaid by subsequent disappointments and traumata—the greater the chances that the therapeutic situation has the potential of becoming similarly rewarding. Conversely, severe deprivations experienced early in life may render the patient chronically impervious to the potential benefits of a benign human relationship. This hypothesis is of course well documented by clinical experience, notably with certain schizophrenic or borderline patients. Ordinarily, these factors are termed transference readiness, or, as I would prefer to call them, susceptibility to therapeutic influence. Parenthetically, it is worth recalling that Freud considered patients suffering from what he called transference neuroses as the most promising candidates for psychoanalysis; in fact, he initially considered the technique contraindicated in all other instances.

2. Capitalizing on the patient's susceptibility to parental-type influences, the therapist initiates a benign, permissive relationship in which the patient is accepted, respected, and encouraged to confide and to communicate directly and uninhibitedly. Thus he is deprived of one set of "defensive" tactics which may be summarized by the statement: How can I trust another person if he continually criticizes, nags, oppresses, corrects, pushes, blames, scolds, punishes, frightens, hurts, or rejects me? In other words, the patient is deprived of his customary "excuses" for fighting a powerful adversary.

In many forms of psychotherapy the creation of a relationship having the foregoing ingredients provides sufficient momentum for a corrective emotional experience. This experience embodies a reduction of guilt; it paves the way toward the abreaction of painful affect; it leads to the exploration and clarification of feelings, attitudes, and values which for one reason or another had been troublesome. Thus, there results an improvement in morale, a rise in self-esteem and hope, and a diminution of anxiety and uncertainty. The key to these therapeutic changes seems to lie in the revival and deepening of a good parent-child relationship which places heavy reliance on the patient's susceptibility to a benign psychological influence. The vehicle for change is suggestibility and the patient's basic responsiveness to loved authority figures. In these forms of psychotherapy the therapist "does" nothing; however, he offers understanding, respect, encouragement, and—most important—a measure of love, all of which may mean a great deal to a person in distress. It is likely that a *very significant amount of psychotherapeutic change occurring in all forms of psychotherapy is attributable to these so-called nonspecific factors which derive their potency largely from their contact with loci of influenceability inherent in the "good" patient.* To the extent that the patient is capable of resonating to the ingredients of a good human relationship, and to the extent that the therapist is able to supply these in terms meaningful to the patient, to that extent therapeutic change may be predicted to occur.

This formulation fully allows for the disappearance or diminution of symptoms such as inhibitions and anxieties which often "melt" in the warmth of love. It is also congruent with this formulation that the "dispensing" or provision of "therapeutic conditions" may be accomplished as readily—often more effectively—by a nonprofessional person. In fact, professional training here has little to offer (except perhaps to mitigate the traditional "countertransference" tendencies in the therapist) and may indeed be detrimental because it frequently fosters an intellectual distance-producing attitude in the trainee.

The foregoing essential aspects of psychotherapy, or for that matter of any healing relationship, are largely synonymous with the nonspecific factors delineated by Frank, [3,9] including prominently: (1) an intense, emotionally charged, confiding relationship; (2) a rationale or myth to account for the "causes" of the patient's distress; (3) new information concerning the "problem" and alternate solutions; (4) attempts to strengthen the patient's expectancy of help and arousal of hope (mediated by the therapist's personal qualities); (5) provision of success experiences which enhance the patient's mastery, competence, and self-esteem; and

(6) the facilitation of emotional arousal. All of these play upon and utilize the patient's suggestibility, defined here as a primitive tendency to yield to social (parental) influence, and they lead to the so-called placebo effects (Shapiro[4]), often confounded with "spontaneous remission" (Eysenck[10, 11]). Stated somewhat differently, the modern psychotherapist, at least on this level, relies to a large extent on the same psychological mechanisms used by the faith healer, shaman, physician, priest, etc., and the results, as reflected by the evidence of therapeutic outcomes, appear to be substantially similar.

As we have seen, the fulcrum on which the therapist's influence turns is delimited by (a) the patient's motivation and (b) his basic susceptibility to psychological influence. These are to some extent definable and measurable (compare the "therapeutic conditions" described by Rogers and researched by Truax and Carkhuff[2]). However, the extent to which the patient responds is probably a fairly idiosyncratic matter, predictable only within broad limits. In the final analysis, the changes achieved in this context are contingent upon the extent to which the patient possesses and has retained the capacity to be a "good," obedient, pliable, conforming, and responsive child. Conversely, to the extent that the patient is lacking this capacity, and to the extent that the motivation to expose himself to a healer's influence is absent, to that extent will the patient fail to avail himself of what the therapist at this level has to offer, and he will experience the therapeutic setting as meaningless and empty. Concomitantly, he will reject the healer.

3. Assuming that the bedrock of psychotherapeutic change is largely coextensive with the patient's basic susceptibility to psychological influence, reconsider those individuals who are more or less impervious to it. As noted earlier, it appears useful to distinguish two groups: (a) individuals who, because of seriously destructive relationships in early childhood or constitutional factors, are seriously deficient in suggestibility; and (b) a much larger group of individuals, ordinarily described as "neurotic," for whom the matter of parental influence has become an issue and who remain entangled in it. Group a, consisting of psychopaths, individuals suffering from so-called impulse disorders, antisocial persons of various kinds to whom societal (parental) injunctions and approval are meaningless, etc., is largely a lost cause for any form of psychotherapy; group b overlaps many "normals" but also comprises the more or less typical candidates for psychotherapy. The basic therapeutic problem here is to undermine or modify the techniques (defenses) by which the patient habitually wards off a healer's psychological influence, and thus to create a condition in

which he can again experience "basic trust." When this goal has been reached, the operations described under (2) can exert their "nonspecific" therapeutic effect.

The application of therapeutic leverage through basic trust

Important aspects of this process have been incisively explored by Haley.[13] A salient example is the therapist's skill in creating a paradoxical situation (called by Haley a benign ordeal) in which the patient is encouraged to communicate with the therapist in "symptomatic" ways; i.e., he is enticed to fight off the therapist's influence in essentially the same way as he had learned to fight off the parents' socializing influence, and when he does so he is placed in a position which effectively makes it impossible to utilize these techniques. Consequently, he is faced with the dilemma of either assuming responsibility for the lack of progress and quitting therapy, which he ordinarily will not do because of the conditions described under (1), or he is forced to modify his usual strategies, which results in therapeutic change.

On a superficial level Haley's analysis creates the unfortunate impression that the therapist is a "manipulator" (in a pejorative sense) who continually engages in one-upmanship maneuvers. Haley also seems to disregard the patient's *motivation* for doing battle with the therapist. In agreement with dynamic teachings, I believe that the most important single factor supporting the patient's "resistance" is his anxiety, the dread of dire consequences (based on fantasy or actual experience) attendant upon the relinquishment of control to the therapist. It is difficult to determine the role of unconscious fantasies about "losing control" in the patient's struggle against the therapist, but I am reasonably convinced that "analyzing" them in and of itself produces relatively little change in the patient. What does produce change is *the patient's realization, on a deep level, that it is futile to fight the therapist with the weapons he has habitually used to control powerful, loved, but potentially dangerous authority figures,* and that these strategies, although "satisfying" in some sense, are basically self-defeating and unrewarding. That is, the patient must realize that the usual controlling techniques at his disposal do not get him what he wants, that what he wanted as a child may not be what he wants as an adult, and that most of his fears are groundless because they are based on erroneous beliefs of helplessness, weakness, and a need to be taken care of, as well as the notion that significant adults are extremely "dangerous."

A case in point is the child who has learned that the parents cannot be trusted to respect him as a person, to gratify his wishes (there is no need to discuss here the distinction between realistic and unrealistic ones), and to protect him, sometimes from his own impulses. As a consequence of such a profound disturbance of the child's security, he becomes devious. That is, he keeps his feelings and wishes to himself, convinced that their exposure would only lead to further humiliation and frustration, and he develops techniques which serve the purpose of (1) providing gratifications while (2) preventing them from being detected. At the same time, the techniques developed in this context express (3) a measure of *defiance* against the parental authority which has proven capricious, disappointing, and painful. The child also typically keeps from himself the intricacies of these maneuvers, of which masturbation, voyeurism, etc., but also other forms of "deviousness" are typical examples. What the child fails to appreciate is the enormous amount of *guilt* generated by what may now be termed a neurotic symptom. The more guilty he feels, the more devious he becomes, but the secrecy of the pleasures also perpetuates the gratifications. Predictably, the process produces progressive estrangement from the parents and social influence. As sketched in this article, an important part of psychotherapy consists of *techniques* for restoring the condition of basic trust.

As Haley correctly points out, a fundamental problem in psychotherapy (and indeed in all human relationships) is the question of *who is in control.* Although couching his operations in very different terms, Freud nevertheless evolved the ingenious technique of seemingly placing the patient in control of the therapist, while in actuality creating for the latter a position of immense power. *It is the judicious utilization of this power which uniquely defines the modern psychotherapist and which constitutes his expertise. The therapist's interpersonal power is deployed more or less deliberately in all forms of psychotherapy regardless of the specific techniques that may be utilized. In other words, if a symptom, belief, interpersonal strategy, or whatever is to change, a measure of external force must be applied.*

To elaborate on the term judicious use of power, there appear to be essentially two ways of "changing" a person's learned behavior: Either the contingencies of the situation force him to change his feelings, beliefs, attitudes, symptoms, etc., or he comes to realize that he *wants* to change some aspect of his personality or behavior. Without wishing to get embroiled in the hoary problem of free will versus determinism, a common-sense statement of the typical neurotic's position is either that he wants to do something but claims he cannot (e.g., a phobic avoidance) or he does something and claims he cannot stop it (e.g., an obsession). In both situations the assertion is made that he has inadequate control over something that he, as well as others, feels he ought to have control over.[2] At this point the orthodox analytic position diverges sharply from learning (behaviorial) approaches. The former asserts that there are "reasons" (motives) for the patient's symptomatic behavior which must be "understood" and that this understanding on the part of the patient will in turn result in therapeutic change. The behavior therapists assert that it is sufficient to change the contingencies and consequences of the patient's behavior, with more expeditious and impressive results. I submit that the differences are more apparent than real. I fully agree with Haley that in analytic psychotherapy, too, the therapist manipulates the situation in such a way that it becomes impossible for the patient to behave in accustomed ways and that the structure of the relationship is such that he is forced to undergo change. By the same token, in desensitization therapy the patient is *forced* to experience graduated doses of anxiety under the guidance of the therapist.

The "insights" which the patient gains in analytic psychotherapy may be valuable in their own right; they may prove rewarding in demonstrating to the patient wishes, impulses, and fantasies whose existence he had only dimly suspected; they may be educational in a variety of other ways; however, they do not change behavior.* In order to change feelings, beliefs, attitudes, and behavior it is crucial to employ techniques which *force* such changes. If the "treatment" is successful, the patient will feel that he has acquired more adequate control, and indeed he has. Thus, it seems questionable that, as far as the abandonment of a "symptom" is concerned, the patient is capable of lifting himself by his bootstraps. (By implication, I assign to "insight" a rather secondary role.)

A simple example will illustrate the point: It is manifestly futile to tell a patient that he can be more trustful of the therapist or less anxious in a given situation. What does help is to *force* him to trust the therapist and sooner or later to expose himself to the anxiety-provoking circumstances. How can he be forced to trust the therapist? In psychoanalysis, he is forced to do so by the (seemingly) simple injunction to abide by the rule of free association; consequently, if he fails to follow the "basic rule," he ceases to be a "good patient" and it is pointed out that he does not "cooperate"

It is interesting to note that some analysts nowadays refer analysands to behavior therapists for the treatment of particular symptoms but continue the "analysis" simultaneously or subsequently. Evidently, they are in accord with Freud's position toward the end of his career that the therapeutic value of psychoanalysis, in the sense of its original goal of behavior change, is severely limited. The aforementioned practice seems to indicate a further step away from Freud's original search for an effective psychotherapeutic technique.

with the therapist. It follows that the responsibility for progress has been thrust into the patient's hands, and he has to struggle with the problem of why he mistrusts the benevolent therapist. In this process he is shown that he manipulates the therapist, keeps secrets from him (see the earlier example), tries to undermine or ignore his authority, etc. He also comes to experience a good deal of anxiety (e.g., fear of censure, loss of love, annihilation, submission, "castration,'). These reactions are demonstrated as being groundless and anchored in erroneous assumptions or beliefs about himself, the therapist's motives, and the world at large. The foregoing strategy also forces the patient to expose, at least in part, the techniques he unwittingly uses to control significant others, many of which are fraught with, and productive of, anxiety.

Trusting the therapist (and significant persons in general) has far-reaching implications. It is indeed a form of submission, a blind faith in the trustworthiness or basic goodness of the other person and an abiding conviction that the other person will not use the power the patient has been forced to place in his hands against the patient except for "therapeutic" purposes. It means, among other things, that in the interest of the patient's maturation the therapist will at times inflict injuries to the patient's "narcissism (his grandiosity, self-will, stubbornness, unbridled wishes), but that he will stringently abstain from embarrassing or humiliating him, and that he will never misuse his power for selfish or ulterior purposes. Thus, *psychotherapy is a series of lessons in basic trust, concomitant with the undermining of those interpersonal strategies the patient has acquired for controlling himself and others.* It places a high premium on open and direct communication, self-disclosure, and a basic willingness (ability) to undergo deprivation, suffering, and self-examination, frequently subsumed under "ego strength."

To repeat: The interpersonal strategies (symptoms, defenses, characterological distortions), insofar as they are not fortuitous maladaptations (e.g., a snake phobia), are techniques for warding off trust in significant others; conversely, the anticipation of a trusting relationship often revives extremely painful feelings of helplessness, loneliness, rejection, domination, oppression, which presumably have led to anxiety and other defensive tactics in the first place. It follows that only in a very restricted sense is the patient reliving the past. Of crucial importance are the transactions with the therapist in the here-and-now. The concept of transference highlights the patient's tendency to respond to powerful authority figures in accustomed (characterological) ways. Accordingly, he tends to fight off the therapist's influence in ways similar to those he had used in fighting off his parents. Thus, *symptoms, at least in part, are techniques of social control* and can be modified if the therapist succeeds in forcing the patient to adopt different strategies or in giving up maladaptive ones.

Problems and implications

One of the basic unresolved problems in psychotherapy as well as in child development is the question of how external control becomes transformed into internal or self-control. Or, how does the individual progress from a state of dependence to a relative state of independence? How does it come about that in some spheres and under some conditions he becomes resistant to external psychological influence, and in other respects remains influence-able, malleable, and open? By what mechanisms do some individuals acquire faulty control over certain physiological functions (e.g., breathing, gastric motility) resulting in the formation of psychosomatic symptoms? Contrary to the psychoanalysts who have proceeded on the assumption that in order to produce significant therapeutic change it is essential to search for "first causes" in the individual's life history, the behavior therapists have produced evidence that it is possible to effect personality and behavior change without recourse to such inquiries. Further, Miller's[14] research has raised the possibility of directly modifying psychosomatic symptoms without delving into antecedent psychological factors. Thus far the evidence is far from conclusive and it would be premature to assert that psychodynamic considerations, including the provision of a therapeutic relationship along the lines sketched in this paper, are expendable in this area.

To some extent control mechanisms are of course essential for social living, and there must be an optimum balance between openness to psychological influence and resistance to it. The psychotherapist, through his interpersonal influence as well as through specific techniques he may employ for modifying certain aspects of the patient's beliefs, feelings, and behaviors, attempts to modify and adjust these control mechanisms which govern the patient's suggestibility or influenceability.

The therapist thus injects himself into the socialization process, and he produces corrections of a "therapeutic" sort. He builds upon the parental authority which in some respects has misfired and paves the way for what Alexander has termed a corrective emotional experience. However, he does more than take the place of a better parent, of a more rational author-ity, or of a better model who provides love, reasonableness, understanding of needs, wishes, and aspirations, thereby correcting the patient's experiential repertoire. In addition, he uses the vantage point of the parental position as a power base from which to effect changes in the patient's interpersonal strategies, in accordance with the principle that *in the final analysis the patient changes out of love for the therapist.* The patient's experience may be formulated as follows: Although it is painful to experience anxiety, give up a symptom, suffer disappointments, abandon stubbornness and grandiosity, have less "pleasure," get along with less approval from others, etc., I will endure these privations because I realize that the higher authority wants me to do these things. More important, the therapist truly has my interest at heart, and by subordinating myself to him I will gain relief from my terrifying loneliness, alienation, and suffering. By subordinating myself to the therapist whom I love and admire (but also fear and hate), I will become like him—share in his strength, fearlessness, maturity, independence, expertness in living, etc. Once I do this, I will have gained the strength to strike out on my own and I can relinquish my struggle with authority figures. I will also have gained the acceptance of society.

It may be seen that therapeutic change thus involves a kind of *trade*— the exchange and modification of one set of (maladaptive) assumptions, behaviors, and strategies for another. This exchange is rooted in, and based upon, the reinstitution of a quasi parent-child relationship, a readiness on the patient's part to endure the reliving (and consequent extinction) of painful experiences, together with the hope that another edition of the parent-child relationship will result in a happier outcome. It must also be assumed that unless there exists a residual memory of benign interpersonal experience, it is not likely that the patient can marshal much hope in therapeutic change. Moreover, unless the therapist somehow succeeds in becoming a loved figure for the patient, his efforts are likewise doomed to failure. Again, the major task of the therapist is to bring about an experience of *trust,* which alone permits him to apply the requisite *leverage* for therapeutically influencing the patient.

The forces sketched in the foregoing are more readily discerned in intensive psychotherapy, but I propose that they are at work—perhaps in attentuated fashion—in any form of psychotherapy, behavior therapy, hypnotherapy, or any other healing relationship. In general terms, the patient trades a symptom or a maladaptive form of behavior for something else, that something else being the love or approval of an authority, even though the latter may be highly symbolic. He will not consummate the trade unless he becomes deeply convinced that the trade balance is favorable for him. The therapist's job is to create the proper conditions, which may vary widely from patient to patient and from circumstance to circumstance.

As Freud well recognized, the ever-present ambivalence, that is, the patient's mistrust, hostility, and rejection of a (parental) influencer, constitutes a formidable obstacle to therapeutic change. The therapist's skill comes to fruition in his ability to ferret out the patient's deepest secrets, that is, the obstacles he unwittingly places between himself and the therapist, and to maximize his opportunities for applying therapeutic leverage.

It is important to recognize that these opportunities occur only inter-mittently and unpredictably. To be sure, as therapy progresses and as his emotional ties to the therapist deepen, the patient's general defensiveness may be expected to lessen. However, the therapeutic strategy must be aimed at making the patient aware of the frustrations inherent in his emo-tional isolation (the tendency to ward off the influence of another person and interpersonal relatedness in general), thereby arousing his affect and intensifying his conflict. When these experiences reach a certain strength, it is possible for the therapist to strike "while the iron is hot." Thus, he is in a position to exert a powerful influence and to have a strong impact on the patient's defenses.

In the above sense it is true that modern psychoanalysis is primarily concerned with the analysis of "ego defenses," *as they manifest themselves in the here-and-now of the patient-therapist relationship,* not with the recall of "repressed" memories or other "unconscious content." To the extent that psychotherapy concerns itself with data in the here-and-now it is, or has the potential of becoming, an empirical science. Reconstructions or the postulation of hypotheses about past experiences that *might* be the "causes" of what is happening in the present may be an interesting intellectual exercise, often quite gratifying to patient and therapist, but they are of little therapeutic value in their own right. They only possibility of effecting therapeutic change lies squarely in what can be forged out of the forces at work in the here-and-now. This assertion seems so self-evident that it should hardly bear reiterating were it not for the fact that it continues to be persistently misunderstood by the opponents of the dynamic therapies. The here-and-now events must be understood and explained in terms of the forces at work in the patient-therapist relationship, major ones of which have been delineated in the foregoing.

The analysis and understanding of interpersonal dynamics in the here-and-now must make allowance for "unconscious" beliefs and assump-tions, fantasies, distortions, body armor, etc., which often govern aspects of the patient's behavior in relation to the therapist (as well as other sig-nificant people in the patient's life). To deprecate or ignore them, as is done by many forms of today's nondynamic therapies, is to grossly underestimate the complexity of human behavior and its determinants. At the present time, it is important to distinguish whether one is studying these forces in their own right or whether one is primarily concerned with producing modifications of specific aspects of the patient's behavior. Freud's notion that the study of these forces and therapy go hand in hand is partly a convenient fiction which has opened the door to interminable therapy. On the other hand, the trouble is that we often do not know whether the dissection of a given belief system or fantasy will result in therapeutic gains, from which it follows that we need to achieve a better understanding of what will pay off and what won't. By focusing on one "problem" at a particular time as opposed to numerous others, the therapist is implicitly making such judgments anyway, although they do not seem to be very systematic. The standard injunction to analyze "from the surface" and "defenses first" vaguely calls attention to the overriding significance of here-and-now events or contemporary forces in the sense discussed in this paper; however, the formulation is far too general to be of real value.

To put the matter bluntly, it is becoming increasingly clear that psychoanalytic writings about technique, although embodying important truths concerning the management of interpersonal forces in the therapeutic relationship, are of very limited value to the practicing psychotherapist. What does the psychotherapist need to know, and what is excess baggage (which moreover has the unfortunate effect of obscuring what he should be concerned with)?

What the psychotherapist needs to know is how to operate within an interpersonal field of forces; he needs to understand the structure and the constraints he imposes upon the relationship and how the patient maneuvers within this field of forces; he needs to have some hypotheses about *why* the patient maneuvers as he does, that is, why he maneuvers in a rigid, maladaptive ("transference") way as opposed to some other way; he needs to *understand* the patient as a struggling person; he needs to be clear about the nature of the influence he can bring to bear on this field of forces in an attempt to modify a significant aspect of the patient's feelings and behavior; he must have relatively specific goals with respect to what he can achieve at a particular juncture and what he may be able to achieve over a period of time; he must have some estimate of the probability of achieving a particular objective; he must understand the forces working against him, not only within the patient and in the therapeutic relationship but also in the patient's total life, toward the end of coping with them adequately; in short, he must be clear of where the patient "lives"; where he wants to go (which may need modification in terms of what, in the therapist's view, is possible and realistic); where he needs to go in order to suffer less (which inevitably engages the therapist's moral and cultural values); and what the therapist can do to help him get there.

What he does not need is constructs such as instincts, ego apparatuses, id, superego, a catalog of defense mechanisms, narcissism, passivity, latent homosexuality, and many others. The utility and value of each concept or construct in current use need to be closely examined for determining its value in the context of therapeutic operations—a task which is long over-due. It may be surmised that as a result of this pruning, a terser and much more concise vocabulary will result. Again, it is of the utmost importance to distinguish between the utility of concepts for therapeutic operations and for other purposes. Thus far, there has been an unfortunate inter-mingling of concepts and therapeutic techniques without much regard for the foregoing considerations.

In earlier communications[1,2] I have called attention to the fact that psychotherapy typically attempts *a variety of tasks,* that these tasks are often quite disparate, and that they may call for very different strategies. They are grouped under the umbrella term psychotherapy because they all involve learning within the context of an interpersonal relationship which assigns to the therapist a position of great influence and power. It seems clear that the "modification" of a particular symptom or behavior is only one of the tasks—and often not a central one—undertaken by the therapist. Nevertheless, the evaluation of therapeutic outcomes—at least in American science—is largely based on *observable* changes of this kind. By the same token, the emphasis of this chapter rests on the understanding and management of interpersonal forces, hence on the development of psychotherapy as a technology. It is undeniably important to move in that direction.

However, as the contemporary pendulum has swung toward the perfection of a therapeutic technology there has been a concomitant deemphasis on the *experiential* aspects of the psychotherapeutic enter-prise. To be sure, these factors have been kept in the foreground by the existential and humanistic forms of psychotherapy, but it is important to underscore their presence in all forms of psychotherapy. I wish to assert that they are present whether or not they are openly recognized or detected by our admittedly crude measuring instruments. Although exceedingly elusive, this component appears just as real as symptom change. Alexander's concept of the "corrective emotional experience" appears to encompass the phenomenon only partially.

Unlike the medical patient whose personality remains essentially unchanged when he is treated for an infection or a broken leg (although here, too, a prolonged or serious illness may have a profound personal significance), the psychotherapy patient, unless the symptom is trivial, undergoes a personally meaningful experience. He not only loses a symptom or modifies some aspect of his behavior, but he often changes his outlook on life, his values, his view of himself. Psychotherapy, especially when carried on for extended periods of time, *may* effect profound changes of this kind. Just as education in the best sense of the term, consists of something other than the acquisition of facts or skills, so psychotherapy may affect the patient in a deep sense. If he is successful, the therapist launches the patient on a different course of life, inculcates some of his own values, fosters self-examination, self-knowledge, and honesty, and participates in the individual's personal development. There are no known "techniques" for effecting such an outcome nor can the outcome be "measured" on a scale or assigned a monetary value.

When Freud abandoned the search for techniques designed to "cure" hysteria and instead turned attention to the life style of the persons in whom hysterical symptoms frequently occurred, he began to forge a tool for the personal development of the individual. His ambivalence concerning psychoanalysis as a therapeutic technique is probably traceable to his inability or unwillingness to draw a clear distinction between psychoanalysis as a treatment technique and psychoanalysis as an educational enterprise. He wanted it both ways, which in retrospect proved impossible. That is, psychoanalysis as a technology for dealing with neurotic symptoms has not proved to be very impressive, and it became a vulnerable target for behavior therapists, whose techniques, at least with certain disorders, are far more effective. Today psychoanalysts, to the extent that they have clarified their goals, tend to lean toward a conception of psychotherapy as an educational process designed to enhance the individual's personal development. Toward the end of his life, this was the position Freud began to embrace.

Even when these goals are raised to preeminence, the objective is still to investigate and mitigate the barriers against interpersonal trust, that is, the entanglements resulting from conflicts between individual strivings and the demands for obedience and acculturation. As these problems are dealt with and resolved, the individual becomes freer to examine his place in the world, to struggle with existential issues, and to evolve his own philosophy of life. In this endeavor he may greatly profit from whatever wisdom, perspective, and insight the therapist has acquired through his own (and hopefully richer) life experience.

Psychotherapy in this sense far transcends conceptions of "behavior modification," and the question of "therapeutic outcomes" as usually formulated assumes a ring of superficiality. The quest for self-knowledge and individuation (in Jung's sense) is a quest for meaning, not for adaptation or adjustment to conditions as they are. In this respect, psychotherapy is revolutionary because it incisively questions prevailing values. Above all, it extols the individual, and, unlike any other human enterprise in contemporary society, persists in the most critical and personal examination of an individual's place in the world.

References

1. Strupp, H. H.: Toward a specification of teaching and learning in psychotherapy. Arch. Gen. Psychiat. (Chicago) 21:203–212, 1969.
2. Strupp, H. H.: Specific vs. nonspecific factors in psychotherapy and the problem of control. Arch. Gen. Psychiat. (Chicago) 23:393–401, 1970.
3. Frank, J. D.: Therapeutic Factors in Psychotherapy. Paper presented at the meetings of the Association for the Advancement of Psychotherapy, New York, 1970.
4. Shapiro, A. K.: Placebo effects in medicine, psychotherapy, and psychoanalysis. In: Bergin, A. E., and Garfield, S. L. (Eds.): Handbook of Psychotherapy and Behavior Change: An Empirical Analysis. New York; John Wiley, 1970, pp. 439–473.
5. Alexander, F.: The dynamics of psychotherapy in the light of learning theory. Amer. J. Psychiat. 120:440–448, 1963.
6. Dollard, J., and Miller, N. E.: Personality and Psychotherapy. New York, McGraw-Hill, 1950.
7. Hilgard, J.: Personality and Hypnosis. Chicago, University of Chicago Press, 1970.
8. Waelder, R.: Basic Theories of Psychoanalysis. New York, International Universities Press, 1960.
9. Frank, J. D.: Persuasion and Healing: A Comparative Study of Psychotherapy. Baltimore, Johns Hopkins Press, 1961.
10. Eysenck, H. J.: The effects of psychotherapy: An evaluation. J. Consult. Psychol. 16:319–324, 1952.
11. Eysenck, H. J.: Behavior Therapy and the Neuroses. New York, Pergamon Press, 1960.
12. Truax, C. B., and Carkhuff, R. R.: Toward Effective Counseling and Psychotherapy: Training and Practice. Chicago, Aldine, 1967.
13. Haley, J.: Strategies of Psychotherapy. New York, Grune & Stratton, 1963.
14. Miller, N. E.: Learning of visceral and glandular responses. Science 163: 434–445, 1969.

Discussion by C. Knight Aldrich, M.D.

This is a provocative paper about an important subject. Psychotherapy indeed needs to make explicit the significant factors in its goals and operations, factors such as the nature of the psychotherapist's influence on his patient. In this effort, almost as important as that of making explicit the outcome of psychotherapy, Dr. Strupp has been and continues to be a pioneer.

I agree with Dr. Strupp that the psychotherapist is a manipulator, whether he plays, by nature or design, the dogmatic, authoritarian parent-martinet or the passive, permissive Great Stoneface. I also applaud Dr. Strupp's insistence on the importance of defining "relatively specific" short- and long-term goals, and on the necessity to differentiate what is important for theory from what is important for therapy.

I am not as satisfied with Dr. Strupp's apparent basic assumption that all infants are essentially alike in their response to "good" mothering, an assumption that leads him to believe that forced regression to a submissive, blind, childlike faith in a parent-surrogate-therapist is always essential for psychotherapeutic change. If there are infants who do not respond positively to traditionally "good" mothering, may psychotherapeutic change for them as adults be possible without forced regression? Indeed, may changes be more effectively and efficiently produced in these patients if they are permitted or encouraged to retain some reservations about trusting their therapists completely and unquestioningly? In these instances, may the effort to force regression, whether successful or not, be contratherapeutic?

Temperament-environment mismatch. Chess, Thomas, and Birch have reported evidence that incompatibility of temperament and early environment is the primary factor in the development of behavior disorders in children.[1] They found two opposite types of biologically determined temperament, one "difficult" and the other "easy," or "slow to warm up," that were overrepresented among children with behavior disorders. They observed that the symptoms demonstrated by these children, resulting from a mismatch between temperament and early parental environment, "are easily misinterpreted as the results of anxiety or as defenses against anxiety."

The "easy" or "slow-to-warm-up" child adjusts easily to his parents, but develops symptoms later if there is "severe dissonance" between intrafamilial and extra-familial pressures. His symptoms can be counteracted by an "opportunity to re-experience new situations without pressure." If, however, the symptoms are not thus counteracted, the "easy" child with unresolved "severe dissonance" may grow up with symptoms which are perceived as the result of conflict and anxiety. He then should fit Strupp's criteria for treatability. (Treatability, in Strupp's terms, requires "the capacity to be a 'good,' obedient, pliable, conforming, and responsive [read 'easy'] child," who will trust the therapist, will learn to perceive the world as the therapist perceives it, and gradually will acquire independence.) In treatment the grown-up "easy" child can be forced into regression, trapped into transference, and then provided with a belated opportunity to "reexperience new (extrafamilial, or socializing) situations without pressure."

The "difficult" child as patient. The "difficult" child, on the other hand, resists parental pressures to alter his spontaneous responses and, presumably on a biological-ly determined basis, shows almost from birth a preference for autonomy over dependency. He never becomes " 'good,' obedient, and pliable." On the other hand, if he learns the rules of adjustment, "from unusually firm, patient, consistent, and tolerant parents," he will learn to "function easily, consistently, and energetically." If, however, he does not have the opportunity to "learn the rules," may he not continue as an adult to suffer from symptoms apparently derived from internal conflict and anxiety? Still unwilling or unable to become a "good, compliant, trusting" patient, he may then be located near the "insusceptibility to treatment" end of any "universal continuum" of psychotherapy that requires patient acceptance of regression. On the other hand, he might be susceptible to treatment that relies on his collaboration in new learning, that avoids forced regression, and that permits him to retain autonomy, or at least the appearance thereof, in most aspects of his life. I can recall, to my embarrassment, 2 patients who in retrospect seem to fit this pattern: one gave up on me after 3 yr. of fighting off my conventional psychotherapeutic efforts to gain her trust and was then relieved in short order by symptom-oriented behavior therapy; the other came to me in desperation after 12 yr. of psychoanalysis with several competent analysts, marked time during 2 yr. of psychotherapy with me, was angry—but relieved—when I went off on sabbatical leave without passing her on to yet another therapist, and attributed her subsequent dramatic symptomatic improvement to modern dance. I think, too, that some patients who do well in group but poorly in individual therapy also belong in this category.

For these grown-up "difficult" children, forced regression to a position of "complete abandonment of so-called defense mechanisms in relation to a healer experienced as possessing superior powers" recapitulates not comforting security, but their unfinished, infantile struggle against their parents, a struggle which persisted and persists whether or not they were given love and encouragement then or love and encouragement now. The temperament-environment mismatch hypothesis requires more validation, but as it stands it needs to be taken seriously in our attempts to understand individual differences in personality development, in the genesis of psychopathology, and in the approach to treatment. Indeed, Dr. Strupp mentions a "biologically determined susceptibility to social influence" early in his paper, but he subsequently appears to write off its import.

Symptom relief. The aims of psychotherapy that does not force regression may well be limited to symptomatic relief. But relief of symptoms is, after all, what most patients are looking for. Personality change, on the other hand, is hard to measure, but in any case, presumably, requires four or five sessions of treatment a week in a prone position for several years. It is, therefore, probably unrealistic to expect personality change of any magnitude to be accomplished in one or two sessions a week over a shorter period of time.

If, then, the goal of psychotherapy (as contrasted with psychoanalysis) is symptom relief, we owe it to each patient to discover and to institute the most efficient and effective pathway available for him to attain sustained relief. How to determine what is most effective is, as we all know, a thorny problem—a problem so thorny that in spite of the efforts of Strupp and many others, psychotherapy is probably the most poorly validated major technique in medicine. What meager evidence there is, however, suggests that short-term psychotherapy, whose practitioners usually attempt to limit regression, may be as effective as its more prestigious long-term counterpart in producing symptomatic relief, and furthermore may be less likely to produce adverse effects.[2]

Secondary gains. One possible adverse effect of long-term or open-ended psychotherapy results from secondary gains of its regressive component. Strupp says that the patient may permit himself to regress if "it promises to liberate (him) from isolation by letting him become a full-fledged adult." However, once an adult who was an "easy" baby can, by assuming the role in therapy of a " 'good,' obedient, conforming, and responsive child . . . , basically trust" a parent figure who is perceived as possessing superior powers, he may lose some of his interest in venturing forth into autonomous activity. In psychotherapy his regressive refuge lasts only an hour or so a week which, according to the theory behind psychoanalytic treatment, gives him too much time to build up resistance against the resolution of those conflicts which keep him from moving toward autonomy. Psychotherapy, by indefinitely offering a taste of regressive security without enough gratification of dependent needs, may perpetuate symptoms by mobilizing hopes for a kind of security that is never realized.[3] The patient's continuing anxiety then may be related more to fear of termination of treatment than to his original conflict.

Summary. In summary, if forced regression puts some patients in a situation which is incompatible with their temperament, if enough regression to provide a base for progression requires conditions unavailable in psychotherapy, and if the secondary gains of the regressive components of treatment can act to prolong both the disability and the treatment process, regression should be perceived as a potential liability as well as an asset in psychotherapy, and at least in some cases should be limited rather than forced.

References

1. Chess, S., Thomas, A., and Birch, H. G.: Behavior problems revisited: Findings of an anterospective study. J. Amer. Acad. Child Psychiat. 6:321–328, 1967.
2. Reid, W. J., and Shyne, A. W.: Brief and Extended Casework. New York, Columbia University Press, 1969.
   Frank, J. D.: The dynamics of the psychotherapeutic relationship. Psychiatry 22:17–39, 1959
   Aldrich, C. K.: Brief psychotherapy: A reappraisal of some theoretical assumptions. Amer. J. Psychiat. 125:37–44, 1969.
3. Harrison, S. I., and Carek, D. J.: A Guide to Psychotherapy. Boston, Little, Brown & Co., 1966.

part 6

RELEVANCE OF PSYCHOANALYSIS TO SOCIAL ISSUES

Is Psychoanalysis Relevant
to Current Issues?

IAN ALGER, M.D.

In May, 1971, a confrontation occurred in Washington, D.C., between 50,000 people, mostly youth, who were assembling to protest the United States involvement in Vietnam, and the Washington police, supported by troops. At the same moment that these two polarizations of power were involved with explosive potential, the American Academy of Psychoanalysis was holding its annual meeting a few blocks from the Washington Monument. More than that, the program topic was "Power and Personality," yet the sessions proceeded without inclusion of the events even then happening in the streets. It was at that time that the Executive Council of the Academy made special provision for the inclusion in the December, 1971, program in New York of a session devoted exclusively to the consideration of the relevance of psychoanalysis to current issues. And since that time, the Council has unanimously voted to encourage the Committee on Programs to include a special session at every future meeting of the Academy.

Psychoanalysis has been challenged increasingly both as a theory and as a therapy. However, what has characterized psychoanalysis throughout its history has been its evolution by the inclusion of newer views as experience and history have presented new insights. Often innovators have been forced to move in new directions as they found a hostile reception to their theories, but above all the essence of the field has been to highlight the importance of the individual and to use the knowledge gained to implement the concepts of human freedom and human dignity.

The early biologically oriented psychoanalytic concepts have been revised, and also new theories have been added which draw heavily on sociology, studies of political process, and system and communication theories. The concept of the relationship between man and his environment has been changed to the concept of the man-environment system, and with this has come the realization of the profound effects of social and cultural factors on the development of personality and the resulting behavior.

That psychoanalysis, both as a theory and as a practice, has relevance and importance in our current world of crisis seems to me clearly evident. However, to meet the challenges not only of the newer psychoanalytic theories, but also of the impending social disasters made vivid in terms of human brutality and suffering, I believe that psychoanalysts must searchingly examine their relationships to themselves, to their patients and colleagues, and to their fellow men in the society at large.

The Honorable Shirley Chisholm will present us with a moving and compelling statement of the current urban crisis as she can so well portray it from her vantage point of those two discriminated-against groups—the Blacks and women. With her statement as stimulus we shall have the views of four eminent psychoanalysts who have focused on the areas of minority groups, women, youth, and education. I hope that this forum is but the beginning of a new tradition in which the Academy will continue the search for greater awareness of human and social conflicts and growth.

A Congresswoman Looks at the Urban Crisis

SHIRLEY CHISHOLM

When the fact that I am going to make a bid for the United States Presidency was referred to earlier, I thought that I heard some slight giggles. Don't be too surprised, my friends, at what can possibly happen. Up and down the length and the breadth of this country today, one finds that there is a great deal of confusion, and a great deal of turbulence, and people go to bed each evening wondering whether or not they are going to be able to see the rising sun when they awake on the morrow, because of what might possibly have happened in their community the night before. Never before in the history of the republic have there been such polarizations of the whites against the Blacks, against the older generations, and in which the Chicanos, the Puerto Ricans, the Blacks, and yes, even the women ask for their own political share of the American dream. I think we must recognize that in spite of the fact that this is a democracy, the so-called American dream has not been fulfilled for thousands of people who still hope that some day that dream may become meaningful and bear substance for them.

One of the problems relating to the future of America's well-being is the crisis of the modern city. Neighborhood deterioration, overcrowded

225

schools, juvenile delinquency and crime, strangled traffic, the war between the city and the suburbs—all are inextricably linked with the prevelant friction between the varied ethnic and religious groups. America's symbol of failure is its cities. Once the cultural heart of America, our cities are quickly becoming places from which to escape. Hundreds of families of skilled and white-collar workers have joined the exodus to the suburbs, and as a result the population of America's major urban centers is becoming increasingly poor and increasingly nonwhite, increasingly uneducated, unskilled, unemployed, and increasingly hopeless. If the goal of our civilization depends upon the tone of life in its cities, this presents a grim augury for America's future. It is past time that the United States prepared itself for a monumental assault upon the crises which have attacked America's urban centers, and success will come only when everything which the ghetto means from a spirtual, economic, social, and psychological viewpoint is finally swept away by a country that is committed to the complete disappearance of inequality. Throughout the nation today public officials are called upon to see that the Black community observes law and order, but almost the entire body of federal, state, and local antidiscrimination laws, and executive orders, has been nullified as a result of nonenforcement, for example, in the construction industry. The growing civil rights crises are directly contributed to by major urban centers that refuse to enforce laws protecting Blacks against discrimination in employment. The time to enforce the law is now, not tomorrow or next year, or at some time in the future. Failure to enforce the statutes by public officials makes a mockery of the law and breeds contempt for it. It is a travesty of law and order.

We do not seem to know what it is that we are trying to accomplish, with all of our milling activity and all of the many programs that we have. We do not like what we see happening in urban America today, but unfortunately we have developed neither concrete goals nor very clear priorities. Among the objectives that we often articulate are revitalizing the commercial centers of our cities, reducing traffic congestion, and eliminating discrimination. All these things sound so attractive, but all too often we find these vague, admirable goals incompatible. These inconsistencies often stem from the fact that in seeking solutions to urban problems we have committed ourselves to specific means before we have committed ourselves to specific goals. A more clearly defined course must be charted if our cities are going to survive. There is need for a new breed of men and women in the professions and in government. There is a need for people who do not cling religiously to the traditional way of doing things when we recognize that that same tradition cannot cope with the kinds of complicated situations that we find in our cities today. We need creators, resourceful and imaginative individuals who can bring a breath of fresh air to the snarled and entangled bureaucratic setup in many of our cities. And these will have to be individuals who can apply modern business and public management techniques and political understanding to the cities problems without getting trapped by outmoded procedures which no longer fit the scheme of today's world.

The urban fiscal crisis has been with us for a very long time. The over-burdened taxpayer no longer has the actual strength to protest or to groan. We need to look very carefully at the whole system of taxation. It is true that cities need money to survive and they certainly need a larger tax base, and not a smaller one. But in the search for new revenue, the cities have consistently turned their backs on an obvious, if politically combustionable, area of relief: tax-exempt property, a traditionally hands-off sector of our economy. Right now the tax-exempt portion of New York City comprises about 1/3 of the city's property valuation. Looked at another way, it amounts to a tax write-off of some 700 million dollars yearly. This field is a very fruitful one for municipal study. There are sound reasons for not taxing hospitals, schools, government buildings, and religious institutions, but in at least two of these general areas, reexamination of existing policy is in order. One is the practice of restricting surplus parcels of city-owned land to church and synagogue use, to accommodate church and synagogue buyers, thus effectively removing that property from public auction and, of course, from future tax rolls. The other is the tax-exempt status enjoyed by such giant public agencies as the New York City Port Authority and the Triborough Bridge and Tunnel Authority. Both have large holdings in New York City, some of which produce income in a normal commercial sense. Their privileged status does not satisfy the needs of the city in the year 1971. This is a new era with new demands and it needs a new philosophy of taxation. Tradition is a poor reason for sustaining outmoded practices. Although this is a politically hazardous issue, these practices need to be revised and carried forward to a new conclusion. The backs of the ordinary taxpayers are being broken daily while millions of dollars that could be utilized slip through loopholes which allow some individuals to avoid the payment of taxes. Cities are powerless to tax without legislative approval and what tax power they do employ is often self-defeating in that it drives middle-class families to seek the tax haven provided by many of the suburbs. The answers to the crises lie with the cities, but the guidelines for major funding will have to come from Congress. The mayors of the large American cities are now reduced to begging for crumbs, and as the flight of the people and businesses to suburbia continues, depleting the central city tax base, the problem is going to get worse.

Added to the great urban crises is the mass of Blacks and Puerto Ricans trapped in debilitating poverty, suffering from underemployment and long-term unemployment. In some cities the unemployment rate has reached that of the great depression of the 1930s. Racism in the American economy is the most persistent and dangerous enemy of the Black and Spanish-speaking populations of the United States. The American Black has peace-fully protested and marched for years, has encountered the courtroom and the seats of government, demanding a justice long denied. The task is to give 20 million Black people the same chance as every other American, most of whose ancestors came here hardly able to speak the English language, but seeking escape from religious, economic, and often political persecution. These people heard of America, the land of the free and the home of the brave, and so they came. Many of them went to night and day schools, acquired skills, became assimilated in the American scheme of things, and moved into the so-called middle class of America. The words at the foot of the Statue of Liberty, "Give me your tired bodies and your wretched souls," meant much to these thousands of people who migrated to this country seeking a haven.

However, the Black people, and the Indians and other minorities, have never been able to pull themselves up by their bootstraps. And do you know why? Because they have never really had the passport to American society, and that passport is a white skin. So often, many of my white friends will say to me, "But Shirley, I'm not rich. My people came over here and they had to work hard." I know that so well. I grew up in the Brownsville area of Brooklyn. I grew up in the midst of a Jewish community prior to my leaving to spend a number of years in the British West Indies, and I can tell you I used to watch the Jewish men and women there behind their pushcarts. I think I see them now, working very hard so that perhaps Joe could become a doctor and mabye Molly a social worker or a teacher. It meant that the older generation really worked to make sure that their young-sters would have an education because to the Jewish people, education is very important. I know that many waves of different ethnic groups had to really work hard to get where they are. But then I turn to many of my friends and say, "Yes, but let me tell you about the group of 50 men in Pennsylvania Station, who retired about 4 yr. ago as Redcaps. These men graduated with Bachelor of Arts degrees in the late 1930s or early 1940s. But when they came out with a sheepskin which was supposed to open the door because they had been educated, their high visibility reared itself at the job interviews, and at the various employment agencies throughout this land, and that sheepskin did not constitute a passport to the American society, which was and is a white skin." So this is something that we may not want to talk about, but we have to face it. We have to face the fact that in America there have been numbers of Black people who have tried to do what the society has said was necessary in order for them to achieve, in order for them to move out into the midstream of American life, politically, economically, and socially. Some have done it, but have encountered tremendous frustrations. Realize that we have never really faced racism, the bugaboo of America which makes us so vulnerable to the attacks of our opponents, both inside and outside this country. The very fact that this melanin, the outer covering of the skin of certain Americans, can cause this land to be in such a state of upheaval today doesn't make sense, because after all when you remove the outer covering, underneath you have the same pair of lungs, the same intestines, and the same blood coursing through the veins. And I dare say that if it were a matter of life and death and it was needed to save any one of us, we would not ask what color the person is. We are going to have to stop generalizing and we are going to have to stop scapegoating and realize that there are grievous ills and inequities in our society. We must have just plain courage to face the issues.

In the cities all over this country, the Black has underlined the crisis because he is shedding the old vestiges of submission, of unending patience, of accommodation. He is imbued with the idea that full citizenship is not marked for delivery tomorrow. The movement of Blacks, Puerto Ricans, and Mexican Americans is not responsible for today's woes, although many people overlook this fact. The influx into cities rather has served to intensify problems which existed back in the days when our large cities were almost entirely white. The human casualties are found in the increased number of people who experience rejection and hostility. The reason lies in the fact that officials and citizens alike have not planned for the future with determination and vision. Our shortsightedness and neglect are particularly evident in housing and education. Many of the programs for slum clearing, public housing, and urban redevelopment intensify the very conditions that they are designed to remedy. Slum clearing increases overcrowding among the lowest income group, segregated neighborhoods have segregated schools, and children are deprived of equal educational opportunities. Immigrants from other lands learned American ways and skills needed for admission to the American middle class and they became assimilated into the life of the community. The color of the nonwhite has remained in this society an almost insurmountable barrier, and color does not disappear.

We cannot rely on gradualism in our country any longer. The fabric of American life is threatened as never before, and the crises of the cities are beyond the scope of any single organization. The stability and prosperity of our cities will depend upon combined efforts because people, just plain people, regardless of their skin color will no longer accept bit-by-bit assurances of human rights.

The decline of our cities has not been an overnight phenomenon. It has been developing for a long time, but the leadership has seen fit to ignore the dangers, thinking that these symptoms would disappear. They did not disappear, and now the entire nation is in panic over the issues of urban crisis, law and order, and other popular sociological and political clichés which are a part of our vocabulary today. There is no doubt in the minds of sensible and reasonable Americans that this nation has been heading for an explosion, fostered by the erroneous belief that a minority in this country would continue to accept being second-class citizens. There can be absolutely no realistic analysis of the recent rioting in northern ghettos for its impact upon the civil rights movement without the prior realization that Black citizens have pressing, long neglected, and just grievances. They do not erupt merely for exercise. They do not curse imaginary obstacles, or practices, neither do they curse imaginary procedures. Their resentment is the raw product of years of prolonged insult and denial. It is my belief that there can be no solution to the urban crisis unless it is coupled with progress through understanding of the race problem, which is the bugaboo of America. If our universities and our churches and all our other social institutions practice discrimination, what can be expected of those who look to them as their guides and mentors? The whole responsibility today cannot be placed on these institutions, of course, because much depends upon the individual's own moral code and his own conscience. For there are many who, although seeing the policies adhered to by these institutions, nevertheless are intelligent enough to pursue the right path and refuse to follow the conventional pattern governing social relationships among people of different races and different creeds.

The problems of our cities will be minimized when America begins to work for true justice—justice in which man will be judged or condemned on the basis of his acts as a man only. America is faced with complex problems, but not unsolvable ones. It is up to her to accept the challenge and face the future undaunted. There is absolutely no more room in America for a "them" and an "us." There is but one America, one citizenship, and one destiny for all, if we are going to survive. Let us hope that we can light a candle of understanding in the hearts of many Americans and realize that all of us must work to create cities in which people *practice* tolerance, *not* talk about it, and live together in peace with one another as good neighbors, working together as equals with dignity. We must find that courage and we must find the heart to get to the roots of the cancer that is destroying our cities.

I learned long ago that it's best to tell the truth and the truth shall set a lot of us free. I don't always expect people to agree with everything I say because we have been exposed to different stimuli. Most of us are the product of our experiences and the kinds of confrontations and situations in which we have found ourselves. I am going to say that the time has come for the professional classes in America to come down from their ivory academic towers and stop dwelling persistently on theory when the whole society is crumbling around us. It is true that there is a necessity for the accumulation of knowledge that one can bring to life's situations, so that we can give leadership a scientific outlook. But the mode must answer the problems of this society, else you will be strangled not only by minority groups but by the alienation of your own sons and daughters, who will not understand what you are about. I can say this to you since for the past 3 yr. it has been my fortune to have visited 43 states in this country, and to have been on some 61 university campuses, because I put speaking engagements at universities first. Many of my peers in the United States Congress don't understand me. They say, "Shirley, you're so crazy, running all over talking to those long-haired kids, not going where the votes are" (that was before the passage of the recent amendment). I realized a long time ago that if there are going to be real changes in America, they will be initiated to a large extent by the younger generation. I do not condone all the behavior of all these young people, because I do not believe in the destruction of life, limb, and/ or property. But one of the things that I have found in the young people in this country, from the most conservative to the most radical, is that they are tired of so much sham and hypocrisy in the leadership of this nation who want the young people to be like them. They are tired of the injustices that they see in America. In their desire to get things done and because of a certain lack of maturity and certain kinds of experiences which would have helped them to approach issues a bit more rationally, they do things that you and I cannot condone. But, they are in a hurry, and we must understand why they do what they do and not use them as the scapegoats for our own failure to make the American dream come true. The young people in this nation did not develop in a vacuum. They are the products of a society which they have watched, in which they have grown up. They have come to learn and to understand what the failures and what the injustices are. So, because so many of them are turning off, I have said to them , "Although I am a 47-year-old Black woman, allow me to cast my lot with you, allow me to see if together we can't work something out."

Our country is in trouble. Our ethnic groups are in trouble. Our youth is in trouble. Many segments of our society are lashing out simultaneously at something or at somebody. Unless we are able to take some hard, stark, naked truths, and digest them, and try to reassess our own values and priorities, and begin to assert our leadership professionally, then all of us will suffer in the holocaust that might take this great nation off the face of the earth. As I travel, I like not what I see, and I like not what I hear. It crosses color lines, age lines, sex lines, and class lines.

I hope I haven't upset anyone unduly, but I think if you understand from where I come, you will be able to accept a few of my remarks.

Relevance of Psychoanalysis to Education

IRVING MARKOWITZ, M.D.

Had psychoanalysis remained truer to some of its early formulations, it would, perhaps, be more pertinent to the current concerns of education. Psychoanalysis, as much as or more than any other movement of its time, gave impetus to the ideas that sanity was freedom; that unreality was the product of bondage; that the reasonableness of behavior should be determined by present rather than past necessity; that it was, indeed, possible for man personally to argue his destiny. The notion that no possibility of action need be automatically foreclosed and that the realm of possibility could be left to personal discretion rather than be determined by family or society was a massive rebellion against the Victorian ethic and a great contribution to human dignity.

Even before psychoanalysis became institutionalized, it had diluted much of its revolutionary promise. The pessimistic view that biology was destiny, the espousal of the medical model of therapy with its implication that love came from the therapist god and did not need to be quantitatively reciprocal, the injunction to therapists that love and therapy must be sold at different counters—whatever other merits these precepts had—were more confining than freeing.

As psychoanalysis aged, it became even more austere and conservative. Freedom was then defined by many analysts as the freedom to fulfill obligation, a paradox with which the Birchites would hardly quarrel. Some analysts, on the basis that identity had to be clearly defined, preferred to see women in skirts, rather than trousers, perhaps because they were still Victorian enough to see the skirt as a possible rising curtain for the arrogant male to disport himself upon the stage so tantalizingly revealed. The concept that identity must wear its own distinctive plumage, that every caste has its own mark, is often an excuse to preserve the status quo. The allocation of fixed segments of time to therapy with the patient often forbidden to know what had gone before in the therapist's life or what was coming after prevented both therapist and patient from establishing continuity of identity. The idea of many therapists that there were correct and incorrect free associations was detrimental to imagination and creativity. The focus on the intrapsychic rather than the social discouraged patients from assailing the unreasonableness of their institutions. Analysts who have stated that dissent is the result of unresolved oedipal strivings or that strong fathers prevent juvenile delinquency—so reminiscent of the alibi for Mussolini that he made the trains run on time—do a disservice to the heritage of psychoanalysis.

Education in recent years has been increasingly concerned with freedom while attempting to maintain some semblance of useful controls. The open classroom, the elimination of required courses, cross-pupil tutoring, class meetings, student involvement in administration, independent study programs, the minicourse, pass-fail grade systems, the one-room schoolroom, cooperative work-study programs, the school within the school, are all efforts to promote greater freedom. These innovations have taken place often in spite of the reluctance of administrators, parents, and the community.

I am presently involved in several educational projects intended to help youngsters who have been unreachable by traditional methods. These are all loose and unstructured projects financed by law enforcement funds. In one of these I serve basically as an instructor in psychodynamics and therapy for relatively inexperienced counselors. This imposes no strain on my credentials or pomposity since their lack of investment in fixed theoretical systems makes them less critical than they might otherwise be. I should like to describe one of these projects at greater length since it raises many questions as to what, if anything, the psychoanalytic perspective can offer to help solve some of our current dilemmas.

This project has taken youngsters from a predominantly Black high school, most of whom had had numerous difficulties with the law, and placed them in a separate wooden dilapidated building adjacent to the high school. The students have had much to do with the rehabilitation of the building. There are no doors to any of the rooms except the bathrooms and, interestingly enough, two rooms intended primarily for use by mental health personnel for testing or interviewing. Learning then is public, but treatment is more or less private. Most of the teaching methods already mentioned are in operation. Students earn unit credits for either self-selected projects or projects decided upon in consultation with their teachers. Failure is measured only by the lack of sufficient unit credits at the end of an as-yet undetermined period of time which will be different for each student. Although there are lecturers who come into the building from the surrounding community to discuss special topics of interest to the pupils, teaching is mainly dyadic, not in the Oxford-Cambridge model, but in the "Eat your cereal" model of home instruction. Many of the youngsters who are unwilling to accept any advice from their mothers are nonetheless accepting this form of instruction from their teachers. Black nationalism has been encouraged by the subject matter chosen for study. The effect on white liberal teachers of encouraging black nationalism and thereby divorcing themselves from their charges is beginning to create some tension in the teachers. Although the pupils and teachers remain close, there are rifts between the teachers and black paraprofessionals and between the teachers and administrators. Some teachers are beginning to ask: Are they bringing the street to the school or the school to the street? Are the pupils becoming a group increasingly involved with one another, or a gang building a hierarchical structure for survival, or both? So far attendance of youngsters who were chronic nonattenders has dramatically improved and some previous nonlearners have accumulated considerable unit credit.

I have been sought out for talks by some students—most will see me only when referred. Although the students seldom haze their teachers, they do enjoy hazing me. I have often been the intermediary between teachers and administrators, also the expert who could soothe the furious parent. The teachers, on the whole, are involved with me. The pupils, on the whole, keep their distance. One student continually solicits my patronage for his candle-making business; another will unexpectedly drop in to see me at the clinic, but basically uses me, as he uses most people, as a safe harbor when other harbors are closed to him. I have defined for the group many of the problems mentioned here. I have solved few of these problems. Yet, there is practically no dissatisfaction with my failure to do so. Both teachers and pupils seem willing to accept me in a relatively inactive role. It is after all their project and I am a guest. Some clinic personnel who insisted on their professional prerogatives found themselves speedily rejected. What I have attempted, not always successfully, is to be available for whatever expertise or friendliness I can offer. I do not know how pertinent I have been to the concerns of these young people. I should like to think that my experience in psychoanalysis has contributed to whatever pertinence I have had.

In its present mood, education is prepared to extend a hearty welcome to those psychoanalysts who can bring their perspectives on the struggle for freedom to schools struggling to deal with freedom's problems and anxieties. If educators cease to foster freedom and its by-products: incentive, enthusiasm, exhilaration—they may be unable to make any lasting dent on the present problems of our society. They may, of course, choose to return to teaching Greek and Latin. If they do, the analysts they will seek as partners are those concerned with sterile insights, regardless of any possible effect on change. Psychoanalysis, whatever its deficiencies, has always maintained its respect for individual worth and has searched diligently for the elusive and unattainable truth, attitudes certainly relevant to a freedom-seeking world. If analysts are to be relevant, they cannot become the Uncle Toms of the repressive Establishment. Not only will they then be irrelevant, they will be used, squeezed dry, and discarded.

Psychoanalytic Theory and Problems of Contemporary Youth

CLAUS B. BAHNSON, PH.D.

The Academy met last in Washington, D.C., during those spring days when young people staged an impressive and intense antiwar demonstration in the Capital, bringing pressure to bear on behalf not only of young people, but of large segments of our population. The Academy, as usual, addressed itself to questions concerning theory and practice, as well as ritual and practicalities of psychoanalysis in the protected conference locales at the same time as thousands of young people expressed human concern and outrage about the inhuman industrial war machinery. The Academy meetings continued also during the ensuing police crackdown and eviction of the young demonstrators, with some of the scenes of police brutality—beating up and molesting of young people—unfolding even in front of the conference hotel.

On this background it was natural to ask, as Ian Alger did: Is psychoanalysis relevant to current issues, or have psychoanalysts become the academic Beckmessers of our society, preoccupied with rules and regulations rather than with main issues of our contemporary life?

My opinion is that, although the clinical practice of psychoanalysis may not have a significant bearing on current social issues, owing to its limited targeting, psychoanalytic theory and its dispassionate concepts

237

have much to offer for our understanding of the current unrest and dis-
quietude and may supply us with both predictions and suggestions of realistic value. Since Freud, many analysts have applied psychoanalytic theory
to social process, e.g., Kardiner, Horney, Linton, Parsons, and others.
I shall not on this occasion attempt to survey their contributions, but simply
point out that the question of the applicability of psychoanalysis to social
process by no means is a new one. Rather, I shall address myself to a brief
description of the kind of youth problems that I have perceived as a teacher
and as a therapist and attempt to apply a few basic psychoanalytic and
ego psychological concepts to these problems.

In order not to be too badly misunderstood when attempting to look
at current youth problems from a historical and theoretical perspective,
let me point out at once that it seems quite apparent that young people presently carry the burden of expressing the malaise and concern of the population in general vis-à-vis the industrial "Establishment,' and that, obviously,
young people express also the concerns and reactions of not-so-young
citizens. The active youth movement decidedly expresses common humanistic and emotional concerns for society at large, and does so with
courage and vigor. In many ways, our contemporary youth, more than
may have been the case in previous generations, expresses the not-so-
conscious needs and desires of their parents, who seem to be caught
in, and controlled by, the system.

Youth's perception of our society certainly is a gloomy one. Young
people perceive society as a mechanical monster, made of steel and glass
and bombs—a meaningless and destructive monster which stands in the
way of individual needs for a creative and meaningful personal life and
destroys that of others. Although there are clear-cut differences by socioeconomic status, this perception decidedly is a leitmotiv among young
people. The goal setting of the Establishment is perceived as inhuman,
destructive, and irrelevant to human and personal needs and is rejected
outright. Thus a young person cannot invest in, and integrate his role within,
this system and must turn away from existing organizations, the usual
educational goals, and the typical challenges of career and economic gain
tackled by the previous generation. Instead, he turns toward goals of
personal expression, immediate and intensive living, sensuality, and often
transcendentalism and mysticism. Young people will not participate in
war or racism and cannot share with the older generation its emphasis on
material values and security.

Interpersonal values also have changed radically. Instead of the classic
monogamic relationship based on continual repression of alternate desires

and impulses, described so well in depth by Sigmund Freud, young people now carry multiple and possibly less charged relationships with other members of small groups within a setting facilitating interchangeability of objects. Hand in hand with this change we also see a change from strictly genital sexuality (with repression of preoccupation with other, developmentally earlier, sexual body zones) to a polymorphous and multileveled sexuality including anal and oral involvement without much restriction or guilt. The taboos of the parents have been replaced with what some of my young patients have labeled "Everything goes." The handling of anal drives also has changed: where the parents defended with ritual, compulsion, denial, and reaction formation, the youngsters act out and let go. In general we have moved from repressive to regressive defenses.

One important aspect of young peoples' adaptation and psychological organization is that they do no longer perceive the relevance of delaying or giving up immediate need gratification in the service of society. Obviously, this observation does not hold for all youngsters and varies by socioeconomic level, region, ethnic background, and so forth. However, the trend seems to me to be rather clear. The reasons probably are twofold: First, social organization has become so complex that even the conservatively motivated young person has difficulty understanding how his effort or input may meaningfully relate to the benefit of society at large. Consequently young people, and perhaps people in general, increasingly adopt a magic outlook concerning social and economic processes, e.g., urban crisis, inflation, size of paycheck, considering them natural phenomena independent of their own behavior. Second, even where the relationship between individual behavior and social process is understood as in the case of the draft or other war-related activities, youth cannot submit to societal demands because it disagrees deeply with the goals to be obtained, and with the ethical and moral orientation of the men in charge of our society. Thus, giving up personal gratification in the service of culture becomes a vice rather than a virtue and young people thus must find their own organized outlets, e.g., peace marches or encounter groups, or must withdraw cathexis completely from the environment and become alienated and narcissistic. The reasons that citizens historically have accepted "civilization and its discontents," as described so vividly by Freud in 1930, is that they could clearly perceive and agree with the reality principle embraced by the society, could understand the necessity of bringing in the harvest, or building a home, or fighting for survival, thus making the necessity for personal sacrifice obvious and meaningful. Freud hypothesized that all cultures are established on the basis of borrowed energy from inhibited libidinal drives and a giving up of undisciplined personal need satisfaction. By and large this analytic principle probably holds. It is when our youth of today cannot see rhyme or reason in the societal demands for their surrender of personal gratification that cultural development as we know it is threatened.

In summary, in our alienated and complex society where no perceivable one-to-one relationship exists between a person's behavior and its potential impact on his society, where the effects for self or for a small group of a given work input are not at all perceivable, there seems to be no reasons for going beyond the pleasure principle or for inhibiting open aggression, other than fear of retaliation and punishment. Young people, particularly in urban settings, perceive society as a magic machine which supplies goods to some and produces destruction and pollution for minority groups here and abroad. This perception is strongly potentiated for underprivileged groups. For these groups, work and the reality principle are particularly difficult to accept because, *de facto,* their output goes to other population groups and to destructive purposes of war and annihilation. Theoretically, there always is conflict between an individual's personal needs for pleasure and existing cultural necessities. Obviously, this conflict is potentiated dramatically when the individual, or the subgroup, does not participate proportionally in the cultural harvest, which is based on his investment in work and his forsaking of primary drives. When the industrial society does not pay him back for his suffering, he cannot identify with the demands, and if society attempts to pay back in substitute currency, such as with mechanical luxuries, a similar situation obtains. Then we see rebellion by minority groups and by youth against the inhuman establishment, coupled with demands for immediate need gratification. One possible sequel of this rejection of restraint and discipline in the service of the society at large may be a sliding back to more primitive social patterns characterized by hedonism and by oral and narcissistic withdrawal coupled with a magical outlook on life.

We may be at such a societal breaking point today, at which some young people are in the process of retreating into an alienated position from which they are unable to influence social process and which, possibly, has a maximizing effect on personal psychopathology. How can a youngster identify with the "ugly [adult] American"? How can he control personal drives and aggression in a setting where the establishment demonstrates a perverse disregard for human suffering and a lack of concern for human dignity? How can the youngster adopt the culture-syntonic ego defenses of sublimation, intellectualization, and displacement, when adult defense mechanisms so clearly appear to him dishonest and as a sham? How can the youngster maintain intense object relations when the object is distasteful and ugly? Why should he not withdraw and set himself more primitive and hedonistic goals?

It seems obvious that young people cannot identify with our current society and its norms and therefore cannot provide the energy necessary for fueling new social developments within the existing system. Because no reason has been given them for not demanding immediate gratification of their needs, they may not, by and large, have available the necessary energy resources to form a strong social dissenting group outside the existing system. The resulting depression and disgust often are undisguised and are available for everyone to observe. Without being unduly pessimistic I suggest that this state of affairs provides a real danger for the continuation of our Western culture as we know it. Historical lessons about the conditions for disintegration of significant cultures should not be forgotten.

Lack of identification in young people with the system makes it impossible for the individual to relieve aggression within the usual externalized projected channels, e.g., the war in Vietnam, or with other displaced targets, and aggression becomes directed within the system itself as we have witnessed it in several ways, e.g., the Panthers, Ralph Nader, unions vs. government, as well as direct and raw violent crime. From the classical condition, under which aggression is directed toward other societies, we have arrived at a nearly undisguised situation of civil war and inward direction of aggression. There is no longer place for displacement of aggression, because the former enemies now have become our brethren, and unification of earthlings has become the long-awaited goal of young people. I presume that the only way aggression could be displaced would be toward extrahuman or extraterrestrial objects under the guise of protecting the human brotherhood on earth.

Because not only the children, but also their parents, are sick and tired of the conditions of life dictated by the industrial monster, parents often support the young who express their own covert longings although they themselves have learned to resign from their needs in order to work and donate their output to society. Industrial society has attempted to appease the personal needs of its donors by producing mechanical objects with symbolic nurturant features: e.g., the luxury car. The older generation has accepted these cultural substitutions for the original drive objects with grace, although with depression. Young people want the "real thing," no longer accept such substitution, and insist on encountering the naked breast rather than the padded dashboard. This is disquieting to the older generation, who somehow perceives the shallowness and failure of the industrial payoff for its own resignation, leaving it empty handed and depressed. Thus, young people do not only reject the aggression and achievement values of industrial society, but also its methods of seduction for work involvement and surrender.

Youth today behaves very much like the child in Hans Christian Andersen's fairy tale "The Emperor's New Clothes." Young people say about the human and technical systems they see around them: "But he has nothing on!" They have the courage to see things as they are on an individual human basis, although, on the other side, their magical view of the monster society does not give them the necessary chance for an effective input. Children not only tell the truth, but they are also both primitive and fantasy bound, and often narcissistic. However, if society could draw on its youth and make use of its refreshing new look at things, we might be able to create alternative forms for living, also involving realistic encounters with production and with the control of environment.

If society does not incorporate and profit from the input of the youth movement, but forces it to remain alienated, regressive, narcissistic, and unrelated, then we are indeed in trouble, and so are the young people. Unless the dissenting young are invited in by those now in power, their only alternative is a withdrawal into a magical world to be supported as an extravaganza by the drab mechanical society, the greater proportion of which then would remain emotionally depleted and hungry for human experiences. One important question then is whether the alienated youth, expressing the covert needs of their elders, can find reentrance into the major contemporary social system so that their experiences and values may modify and put a stop to the existing disintegration and disarray of our society. If the young cannot find entrance, they will have to burn the bridges and remain as an externalized and dangerous drive representation of the repressive society, very much as was the case with the attractive witches who were hunted and burned because they represented the forbidden longings and desires of their persecutors.

I very much hope that it will be possible for us to listen carefully to what young people express and to prevent a premature rejection of their imagery, thus also preventing their own destruction as well as the deterioration of our society.

at which they have been taught to fear most, that of being
e." Perhaps even more basically, they fear loss of the possibility
to other people. If they do not fulfill the stereotypic role, they
ay relinquish the only basis on which they will be allowed
others. They are threatened with being alone, isolated, and

atively, many women suffer deeply from the sense of failure,
at they have developed no ability that is valued by the larger
thing to which they are committed, nothing they can do well.
rced to cling to a husband to achieve any sense of value, or to
en, often using many covert actions psychologically destructive
sband and children. Women must therefore constantly try to
to accommodate to others, and many resent doing so. Open
of resentment would threaten their position. After a long buildup
sed resentment, its expression would seem excessive even to
themselves. They then might further disparage themselves
reby deepening the cycle of feelings of unworthiness. All this
follows from the basic premise of prescribed compliance and

are many more aspects of women's dilemma which could be
. Women are now trying to break out of some of these binds.
so they are clearly going to come into conflict both with individual
ith the dominant social mores. The situation is further compound-
fact that women are seeking to develop an enlarged vision for
precisely at the time when society has no need for this at all—
civilization as a whole also enlarges its concept of what it values.
it needs the talents of all its people in many areas—health,
housing, etc. But these needs are not presently endorsed.
rief dip into some of the problems of women indicates some of
ew areas which psychiatrists should examine. For each of the
ups of "unnecessary people" the prolbems are different because
ent history and set of circumstances. The development of all the
ary people" would clearly seem to lead to conflict with the domi-
ls in our civilization. How are we as psychoanalysts to view this?
areas are important. Conflict, which is inevitable, is after all
ur psychoanalytic areas of expertise, especially in making
onflicts which are unrecognized but powerful. We have not,
encompassed an understanding of conflict of this order. One
ditional beliefs has been that conflict need not be feared and that
ings can cope with it.

Women and Other "Unnecessary People"

JEAN B. MILLER, M.D.

Erik Erikson, one of the leaders of our field, has written, "The special
dangers of the nuclear age clearly have brought male leadership close to
the limit of its adaptive imagination. The dominant male identity is based
on a fondness for 'what works' and of what man can make, whether it
helps to build or to destroy. For this very reason the all too obvious necessity to sacrifice some of the possible climaxes of technological triumph and
of political hegemony for the sake of the mere preservation of mankind
is not in itself an endeavor enhancing the male sense of identity . . . . Maybe
if women would only gain the determination to represent as image pro-
viders and law givers what they have always stood for privately in evolution and in history, they might well be mobilized to add an ethically restrain-
ing, because truly supranational power to politics in the widest sense.

"This I think, many men and women hope openly and many more
secretly. But their hope collides with dominant trends in our technological
civilization and with deep inner resistances as well."[1]

Erikson touches on one kind of hope. Women today have many others
too. But what does happen when people's deep hopes—and needs—
collide with dominant trends in our civilization, and they meet with deep

243

inner resistances? This would certainly seem to be the business of psycho-analysis. It requires discussion of other trends in our civilization in addition to the nuclear threat.

Parenthetically I would differ with some of Erikson's emphases. For example, women need to develop their concerns if they are important to women, not in order to save men from their current impasse. In so doing they may well create a counterforce to some of the dominant male values, but this should not be their primary intent. Erikson's formulation may be an example of one of the many, often subtle ways in which even the most generous and humanitarian of men see things, of course, from a male point of view. Also, current male identity is based on more than a fondness for "what works." That topic would require a long elaboration.

One characteristic of our current civilization seems to be new and of overwhelming importance for a large segment of our people, in fact the majority: our civilization does not need or value them. The central productive operations of our highly industrialized society do not need the participation of anyone outside of the mainstream of adult white men. All other groups are really not necessary to the productive enterprise. Indeed, they are a drag to be somehow handled in the cheapest possible way. These are the minority groups, the youth, women, and the elderly. They are all relegated to the marginal service functions at the lowest possible pay and esteem, or to no function at all. In the latter case they are to be salted away at the least cost—the minorities on welfare, the youth in ever-extended, often unnecessary schooling, women in unpaid labor at home, and the elderly in the most shameful of conditions.

All these groups evidence symptoms of the fact that society does not find them necessary or important. So, for example, a new book on drug abuse among the youth elaborates the premise that drug use reflects young people's deep sense that they are not needed or valued.[2]

In addition, our efficient economy has now produced crises in all of the "living arrangements" that industrial civilization itself has created. It produced cities, and the cities are now in crisis. It produced universal education, also in crisis. It led to the nuclear family but the family is in crisis. The same applies to modern medicine, housing, transportation, and all the rest of the environment.

To complete the circle, the "unnecessary people" are the people who are the first and the hardest hit by these crises. In cities, it is the minorities and other poor who are first affected; in education, the minorities and the youth feel the impact; in families, the young and the women are the first to experience the crises directly. These groups have therefore been the ones

to react openly—the minorities, the y
not only are the reflections of their pa
of the dilemmas of our total civiliza

These are obviously problems o
same way if we had not first arrived
at least, certain ideals of equality and
to his own full development. We nov
have incorporated some of these
themselves.

The solutions to the problems of c
not immediately apparent. It seems
analysts are to work with any mem
people, they will have to develop a c
the pervading sense that society does n
ment or participation.

A brief mention of women's cur
some of the problems. Until now won
that their major developmental goals
interests of other people. I can't imagin
of normality which stated that the goa
needs of another person to the negle
has been the implicit, if not explicit,
development.

Women's lives have been organize
men's needs, as men defined them. (T
needs, e.g., the need to feel dominant in
to aim first and foremost, to fashion her
able and attractive to men. If she s
(and sustains it), she may then go on
in other ways as well. The implications
ment are endless and bear directly or
disturbances in husbands and children

Clearly, women's development ca
these narrow bounds. Women have n
fulfilled within this restricted framewor

Of course, there are many differe
development who desire different things
point. Women are not all the same and a
Some fear success in intellectual or oth
disrupt a deeply imbued conception of wl

up the t
"unfemir
of relatin
feel they
to relate
unrelatec

Alte
knowing
society,
They are
their chil
to both
please ar
expressic
of suppr
the wom
for it, tl
and mol
submissi

The
elaborat
As they
men and
ed by th
themselv
unless o
Obvious
educatio

Thi
the vast
other gr
of a difl
"unnece
nant tre

Tw
one of
explicit
howeve
of our t
human

Second, we are faced with the challenge of enlarging our theoretical outlook in order to understand irrationality in a new way. All the "unnecessary people" are receiving the message that their full development is unneeded and unwanted. For anyone in our culture today this must constitute an irrationality that he or she cannot accept.

One way of looking at psychoanalytic theory is to view it as an attempt to explain the unproductive, repetitive irrationalities in which people can become ensnared. Psychoanalysis gave us the first theory and methodology for investigating and changing some of the human irrationalities which had previously seemed so inexplicable and immutable.

One pivotal point around which psychoanalytic theory has subsequently revolved is the delineation of the source of these irrationalities. Do their origins lie in derivatives of biological characteristics inherent in human beings or in the environmental irrationalities to which the individual is subjected? It seems clear that the major irrationalities with which people today contend derive not from their inner biological drives but from the larger societal context. Certainly this is true for the majority of people, "the unnecessary ones."

References

1. Erikson, E.: Inner and outer space: Reflections on womanhood. Daedalus, pp. 582 606, Spring, 1964.
2. Rosenthal, M. S., and Mothner, I.: The Three Way Connection: Drugs-Parents-Children. Boston, Houghton Mifflin, 1972.

The Problems of Minority Groups

ALBERT E. SCHEFLEN, M.D.

Inasmuch as the biggest problem of minority groups is the majority group, we must start this discussion by talking about larger social, political, and economic scenes in America. All of us have come under a system of increasing constraints, political economic, and epistemological. But those of us who do relatively well and enjoy some measure of influence or power do not adequately use this to defend the common good. Instead we tend to turn on those below us in the hierarchy and impose on them a further series of constraints.

Some general constraints in the American social order

We can distinguish three levels of control on the people of America. At the lowest level general control is maintained by the political structure of local, state, and federal government. The first of two mechanisms of political control which seem to be increasing in America is semantic distortion. It is now *usual* for governmental officials to call all hearts spades and all spades diamonds. Military aggression is called defense; racism is called law and order; and so on. There is nothing new about this and we are all

249

aware of it; yet the practice continues and seems to be effective. One reason for its success in the tendency of Americans to give an almost magical status to words and names. Thus rhetorical statements *about an event* are accepted as if these statements were the event. Another reason for the effectiveness of semantic distortion is the number of highly intelligent American scientists and artists who are willing to commit their careers to the practice.

A second ominous mechanism of political control in the United States is the tactical use of assassination. As a consequence of this tactic, minority group leadership or leadership for change is continuously ravaged. Many liberals and radicals believe that King, the Kennedys, Che Guevara, and other leaders were assassinated by the CIA or by some other governmental agencies in a conspiracy. I do not, of course, know whether these charges are justified; but the point is that *it is not necessary in the United States to conspire for assassination* because mechanisms for assassination are built into a culture of violence. There are hundreds of thousands of armed men in America who feel justified in killing a political opponent or a person of different color or ethnicity, and need little excuse to do so. In this climate a key official need only make an insinuation about some opponent or rebellious faction and his following will take it from there.

The Kent State massacre is an example. With an armed National Guard on the scene and anger running high, the governor of Ohio and the head of the National Guard appeared on the media and hinted that violent suppression would be justified. The next day a number of guardsmen did the trigger pulling. Then, in typical American fashion, legal proceedings were instituted to blame the victims. For these reasons I am today concerned for the safety of George Meany. He has finally roused himself out of a 20-yr., Rip Van Winkle slumber and taken a strong stand against the Nixon administration, whereupon Connally appeared on television to declare Meany an enemy of the state. Interestingly enough, Connally used the term arrogant—a term which is usually used to finger a Black protester.

The concept of paranoid thinking plays a key role in this kind of politics. If a person or faction charges an establishment with conspiracy when in fact no one has actually *said* an assassination should be committed or when no one has actually been hired, those who make the charge can be said to be paranoid. This charge usefully conceals the fact that a chain or unconscious or covert communicational relations has had the same consequences as an overt conspiracy.

The psychiatrist can play a pivotal role in this kind of political machination. He can diagnose the protesters as paranoid on the technicality that no overt conspiracy can be identified or he can point out that the charge may be overly literal but also that it may be based upon a hidden sequence of events. In short, the clinician must constantly ask himself for whom he is working.

But major control in the United States is probably at a higher level than government. It is difficult to continue the illusion that the Federal government is anything more than an agency for the powerful corporate oligarchy which runs the affairs of the nation. I think it is no longer possible for an administration to oppose the dictates of this oligarchy and it may no longer be possible to elect a president who does not suit the interests of the military-industrial complex. Thus many liberals complain that the Nixon administration does not stop the bombing of North Vietnam and the war in general. But I think he lacks the power to call an end to this very profitable venture even if he wanted to.

We came to this sort of economic dictatorship by a series of steps. In Roosevelt's time the ethnic groups and union members were encouraged to consider themselves honorary members of the WASP Establishment and they actually came to regard themselves as having such prerogatives. Subsequent events provided the working man with ample consumer goods and television, which keep him quietly at home. Eisenhower was probably the last President who had the popularity to stand against the economic oligarchy. He warned us about the military-industrial complex but he did not take a stand on the matter.

This economic power structure has a vast supportive base. Continuous warfare not only provides millions of jobs but keeps many young people off the labor market. The abundance of material conveniences and a belief that each working man is *in* the Establishment brings a majority of Americans within one of the two major political parties. The pretense of choice in an election and the ability to change one administration for another almost identical one preserves the illusion of democracy. And Americans are preoccupied with political rights so they think they are not controlled as long as they have the right to speak and vote. Thus, we Americans say that China and Russia are totalitarian because control is exercised by *political* suppression. We are not oriented to the politics of economic control so we fail to see its effectiveness or we even regard it a good thing.

A third kind of control which entraps the middle class in America is epistemological. In the tradition of Western thought we hold to the myth of individualism. We sustain the myth by almost compulsively exercising minute and trivial differences in speech content, dress, food styles, and the like which we then point to as evidence that vast individual differences occur. When we do experience the constraints of the social order we can automatically deny our conformity by using a cliché to reaffirm our individuality. We say, "I am an individual. I am an individual. I am an individual." (Those Americans who have not learned to say this phrase in the face of conformities can learn, for a fee, how to do so.)

In middle-class America the myth of individuality ordinarily refers to freedom from the domination of parents. It is thus achieved by breaking away from the family and entering upon the upward-mobility ladder. Thus the immigrant or mobile working-class citizen trades his family and peer group affiliations for membership in a corporation or in some other institution. The mobility he thus acquires makes him more useful to industry or to the military for he can transfer easily and attach his loyalties to his job. But he may have made a mistake in trading in his cultural and peer group membership. Maybe he can now curse, masturbate, or marry a Catholic against his mother's disapproval but he will not acquire freedom of behavior or ideation as a member of the middle class and its institutions. And he certainly will not find individualism as a corporate executive, as a university professor, or as a member of the AMA or of a psychoanalytic society.

In short, the dream of individualism has been turned around for use as a recruiting slogan and a carrot to induce us to give our loyalty to middle-class institutions and keep us at our workbenches.

The belief in individuality can be turned against us in yet another way. If we can believe in self-determination by personality and effort, we can be captured by another old Western myth. *We can believe that individuals cause the problems of larger social systems. Then individuals and factions can be blamed for problems which are beyond their control.* The fear of being so blamed constitutes a major way of controlling human behavior. And the exercise of blame in scapegoating can be used to exclude or get rid of those who are undersirable and to cover up in the process the problems of institutions and governments.

We can all identify with the experience of being controlled by such an epistemology. We start life by being charged with having bad seed, original sin, or instincts. And we strive hard in conformity to get over these evils. But we do not escape the possibility of being blamed, for our guilt is not the essential element. It is rather the politics of institutional control in use, at all levels from the family to the United Nations.

This reductionistic notion—that individuals are the cause of systems problems—costs us heavily in another way. It can lead us to a preoccupation with our own psychological processes in an endless search for insight when often we need an "exsight"—a better understanding of contexts and ecosystems. In fact, it should be quite easy to exercise economic and political domination over a people who examine only their own navels and blame themselves alone when they are in troubled times. A large segment of middle-class American has been copped out this way for the last 2 decades.

This point is not to disparage the tactical value of insight in psychotherapy or in everyday life. It is a critical tool of our life experience to examine our role, to observe our behavior and determine our thoughts and feeling in any situation. And many of us have to learn how to determine those aspects which have not been conscious to us. But we must not use a tactic as a total life strategy. Eventually a psychoanalytic patient must move beyond the tactics of "self-examination" to apply what he has learned to the broader experiences of his life. And as citizens we must examine our own motivations but we also look about us, for the world is not merely a projection of our cognitive experience or a consequence of our motivations.

Some mechanisms in the hierarchical control of minorities

So far I have sketched a thesis something as follows: the political structure of the United States has fallen into the service of manipulations which are advantageous to a powerful military-corporate oligarchy in which the citizenry is copped out in blame systems, reaffirmations of individualism, and other exercises in psychological rumination.

Liberals and radicals in the United States protest this state of affairs but a majority of middle-class Americans appear to support and justify it. The working-class white protests vigorously, but he blames the minority groups for this plight and rather complacently accepts the present political regime and the corporate oligarchy. In short, the remarkable phenomenon of contemporary America is the passing of blame *down* the hierarchy from the middle class and working class to the minority groups. This direction of protest constitutes a complete about-face from the 1930s when the working class blamed government and big business for its difficulties. This direction of scapegoating is reminiscent of the situation in Nazi Germany.

In short, the middle- and working-class majority in America and the old ethnic groups, themselves victimized at higher levels, tend to turn the mechanisms of suppression upon minority group members. We can consider this matter a mere question of racism but there is much more to the matter. Minority group members constitute a cheap source of labor and do not have to be kept on the payroll or given fringe benefits. And the politicians find appeals to racism and the scapegoating mechanisms useful. So we cannot explain away these problems with simple statements about the psychology of prejudices. Furthermore we should interest ourselves in the actual behavior by which hierarchical suppression is maintained in America, not merely with the motives for doing so.

I shall briefly outline three major mechanisms of minority suppression that have interested us in our territorial studies in New York.

Tokenism. The first is the selection of a few minority group members for admission into middle-class life and middle-class establishments. This practice is often called tokenism. This term pays heed to the political usefulness of offsetting laws against discrimination by having a few minority group members conspicuously placed in white establishments, but there is more to the matter than this. *The recruitment of the most able minority group members into the establishment provides a continuous brain and leadership drain of the minority group communities,* and most minority group members who "make it" leave their old neighborhoods and causes and may even become discriminators themselves. In short, when an ethnic majority provides opportunities for selected members of a minority group, the ethnic minority as a whole may suffer.

The answer is not to continue discrimination and separatism so that no Black or other minority leadership can make it in the middle class. But this dilemma exists only because *the price of a middle-class income in the United States demands a renunciation of one's original cultural identity and affiliation.* Each immigrant group has paid just that price for making it into the bottom of the middle class. The solution will await a time when this society can accept a higher variance in behavior from its citizens, a real individuality instead of a platitudinous, rhetorical one.

But the political aspect of tokenism is not to be ignored in this analysis. It becomes evident in traveling around the United States that more Blacks and Spanish-speaking people hold Establishment positions than was the case a decade ago. But the statistics belie the idea that Black peoples are better off. Although Black incomes have risen in the last decade, they have risen more slowly than white incomes so that *the discrepancy in earning power is greater now than it was in the 1950s.* Although the government says unemployment is at about 6 percent in the United States, it is 25 to 30 percent in the inner city. Although more Black men graduated from medical school in 1970 than ever before the ratio of Black physicians per hundred thousand population is not larger than it was in 1910.

Ethnic encirclement. The second mechanism of minority group containment is based on an analagous illusion. The United States has passed laws against discrimination and can show proof as it were that its government does not engage in discriminatory practices. *But it does not have to engage in such efforts, for the minority groups of the urban United States are contained within concentric rings of old ethnic peoples. Members of these ethnic groups do the battling and suppression for the society as a whole.* So effective is this mechanism that the mainstream middle class rarely has to bare its discriminatory fangs and can even pretend not to have them. But in case you believe this myth, witness what happens when a determined governmental administration does occasionally try to build a minority group housing project in a middle-class neighborhood as the Lindsay administration did in Forest Hills. Then one sees the professionals and eggheads screaming with red necks on the picket lines of protest.

The encirclement of minorities in the inner city by a ring of old ethnic peoples is a pattern of residential territoriality throughout America. In the Bronx, for example, the central region is almost entirely Black and Puerto Rican in a cone-shaped inner-city ghetto stretching north from Harlem. To the east, west, and north, groups of Italian, Irish, and Jewish working-class peoples defend their turf against further minority group migration with vigor and determination. To the far north in Westchester and Connecticut live the upper-middle-class peoples who control Manhattan. They can pass under this battleground by subway or around it by expressway. Thousands have commuted every day for decades between Manhattan and Connecticut and have never seen a ghetto.

The same principle of containment holds for occupational as well as for residential territory. In New York the lower-echelon public servants are of the older ethnic minority members. Each ethnicity holds control of one or more occupational domains. The Italian Americans own sanitation, for example, whereas the Irish still have the police force and the Jews have local civil service and secondary education.

This is the very occupational turf which upwardly mobile Puerto Ricans and Blacks invade. The old ethnic groups try to defend these positions and a great deal of bitterness results. This was the central issue in the New York school strike; ethnic groups who were themselves discriminated against or even treated to genocide a generation ago are now in the position of being racists. But they are graciously helped in their conflict about these matters by an "insight" that it is minority groups who threaten the social order; it is welfare, not war, that causes inflation. A multimillionaire WASP who lives in Connecticut was recently elected senator in New York by winning the support of white labor with the slogan "Isn't it about time WE had a senator."

As long as the ethnic minorities of America are divided against each other in this kind of frontier warfare, the economic and political power structure of the United States has nothing to fear. The 1960 uprising by the white left and the Black nationalists was hopelessly outgunned and outmaneuvered. President Johnson, for instance, was forced by public opinion to discontinue the bombing of North Vietnam 4 yr. ago, but the present administration can bomb for days on end without even bothering to launch a propaganda campaign of justification. Ethnic divisiveness and containment are possibly the critical factor in current American political and economic control.

The use of scientism. The majority group in America participates in one other way in class and minority suppression by using selected fragments of scientific explanation in a political way. Few do so wittingly, of course, for each doctrinal school in the sciences of man recruits and indoctrinates advocates who deeply believe the part truths of that particular approach. From then on, if their views or findings turn leverage for or against any particular group of people the results are automatically political.

This mechanism is based on the scientistic fallacy of reductionism which lies deep in Western and Aristotelian thought. In reductionistic approaches it is believed that some of the many determinants of human behavior are the real, true, deep, or important ones, whereas the others are false or unimportant. This kind of preemptiveness has been the curse of psychoanalysis, in that instinct theories have been regarded as the "real" explanations, whereas cultural, social, economic, or other theories have been held to be superficial. But all the classical, presystems sciences have played this status game.

Psychoanalytic or any other thought which features motivation, drive, cognition, personality, instinct, or any other intraorganismic process as *the* cause of human behavior tends thereby to ignore or deemphasize ecological explanations. *Thus psychoanalytic, genetic, and any other organismic approach to human behavior can be used politically to support the practice of blaming poverty peoples and minority peoples for their lot in the social order.* Whenever it can be established that the reasons for economic, social, cultural, and ecological states lie within the people, it can then be stated or implied that the origins of these conditions *do not* rest within the social order as a whole. It can be claimed that having too little money has to do only with motivation or personality and not with the fact that other people have too much money. It can be held that garbage in the streets of the ghetto is a consequence of the behavior of minority group residents and thus denied that white sanitation teams do not go into ghetto streets. It can be held that Black houses are run down because of the character of their residents and denied that run-down houses are rented to Black people.

If the psychoanalyst generalizes from his experience behind the couch and his predilection for psychodynamic explanation to the social problems of his day, he may say that the problems of minority peoples stem *from the nature of minority peoples.* In this case the psychoanalyst is blaming the victim. He is supporting the present system of hierarchical control and discrimination whether he realizes it or not.

The same must be said about the researcher. If a researcher makes open political statements, as I am doing here tonight, he will be criticized for being a politician. But when he produces statistics or generalizations which support *existing* myths he does not see that he is acting in a political way. Thus, when Jensen produces figures which seem to show that Black IQs are lower than those of whites *and explains this on a genetic basis,* he is acting politically. He is ignoring the fact that the IQ test measures, in part, the products of middle-class education and the fact that education is discriminatory in the United States. But he is surprised when people say he is acting politically.

But Stokely has no such scruples or naïveté. He uses Jensen's data and his status as a Nobel laureate to support his notion that Blacks are racially inferior and therefore cannot be educated. They should therefore be trained, he claims, for menial jobs or be paid to allow their own sterilization. *Whatever a clinician's or researcher's motives his results will be used politically, so it is his personal responsibility to predict this eventually.*

The role of the psychoanalyst

A number of psychiatrists and psychoanalysts have been willing to use the prestige of psychoanalytic or psychodynamic theory for political leverage. Six years ago 500 American psychiatrists were willing to pervert their clinical skills to declare that Goldwater was paranoid or mentally ill. Nowadays some speak of the psychopathology of the youth movements. Others ascribe the lot of minority peples to their personalities or motivations without regard to the sociocultural and economic aspects of poverty discrimination and ghetto life. To do this is to foster the political tactic of blaming the victim.

Such political uses of psychoanalytic theory should stir organized psychoanalysis to at least a disclaimer. So far, however, the movement has remained silent and our organizations have tried to avoid an airing of the issues.

Experiments in Advocacy Research

ROBERT JAY LIFTON, M.D.

I want to take the liberty of indicating my sense of this award by quoting one of my bird cartoons, in which a bird is looking up hopefully and saying naïvely, "All of a sudden I had this wonderful feeling: I am me!" The other bird—appearing more jaundiced, experienced, and cynical—looks down and says, "You were wrong."

I do appreciate the spirit of this award since, as Dr. Bieber stated, it reflects a strong concern for social issues. I might mention another of the bird cartoons which provides a commentary on our field. In this cartoon the first bird, again looking small and hopeful but scared, says, "I'm afraid of the world. There's something dark about it." An older, taller, more knowing, and slightly pompous bird looks down and says, "That's just your imagination, my child."

That comment reflects much of what we do in psychiatry: we recommend new ways, but get stuck in old and limiting definitions of ourselves.

This chapter is the William V. Silverberg Memorial Award Lecture given by Dr. Lifton on presentation of the award to him at the December, 1971, meeting of the American Academy of Psychoanalysis. Copyright © 1972 by Robert Jay Lifton.

I see advocacy research as one attempt to break away from these old patterns. Advocacy research, or advocacy psychiatry in general, is something evolving on many sides. It is an idea whose time has come, or almost come. Obviously it has to do with avoiding the usual separation of the issues that we study and the people that we treat from a larger social sphere.

Advocacy psychiatry has to do with a simultaneous commitment one makes to social and historical forces and groups. The advocacy lies in combining professional tradition with a critical stance toward both that tradition and the more general ethical and political status quo.

The investigator's own subjectivity, his own sense of himself in process, has also been very important in this kind of approach as it is in other forms of psychohistorical work. We often speak of "disciplined subjectivity." It is not clear who first used that term—Margaret Mead and Erik Erikson are two distinguished claimants, so I certainly would not add my claim to it. But there is an increasing movement toward putting one's subjectivity, as the young now say, "out front."

There are two prevailing modes or models in the kind of psychohistory we are evolving. One of these models is Erikson's fundamental contribution, "the great man in history," in which the biography or psychobiography of the great man as it occurred *in* history is studied. The breakthrough of the individual, the great man, is seen simultaneously as a source of his own health and growth on the one hand and of those of his culture or his people on the other. In Erikson's model the great man is seen as one who cannot solve his own problems without solving larger historical ones at the same time. In the other psychohistorical paradigm, the one in which I have been involved, one studies intensely a group of people who have been through a particular historical experience and tries to find common themes in their responses and their innovations. In both these kinds of psychohistorical work one really must use the self as an instrument. I found myself doing precisely this in various research endeavors without being aware of it.

For me the key personal event for this issue of advocacy research was my pivotal experience in Hiroshima in 1962. To learn something about the psychological effects of the first use of the atomic bomb I had to involve myself deeply in the ethical dimensions of the event, and I had to make this ethical involvement clear to the people I wished to study. As it turned out there already was an American medical group in Hiroshima doing studies of the physical aftereffects of the bomb. This group, the Atomic Bomb Casuality Commission, had been, and still is, sponsored by the Atomic Energy Commission, which meant that the organization studying medical aftereffects was supported by the same organization that carried out nuclear testing. The people of Hiroshima have been quite conscious of this, and it has been a kind of Kafkaesque situation for them. Their feelings about the Atomic Bomb Casuality Commission were, to say the least, ambivalent. I realized that it was also a kind of Kafkaesque situation for me, an American psychiatrist, to be investigating the psychological effects of the bomb. What I was doing, after all, was asking the people of Hiroshima: "How do you feel about that bomb we dropped on you 17 yr. ago?"

The result of all this was that the pragmatic needs of the research, getting the cooperation of the people I wanted to work with, forced me to examine my own ethical relation to the work. As I delicately approached people in Hiroshima I found myself not only emphasizing my intellectual independence, my being a nongovernmental scholar, but also stating very clearly my own ethical motivations for the research. I told people that I was doing this work because I was concerned with peace. I had been involved in the early academic peace movement, and an article I had written on nuclear weapons and the Japanese peace symbols had been translated into Japanese; so my statement had some credibility. I told people that I was conducting this research not (as they feared the Atomic Bomb Casuality Commission was doing) to find out how to deal with casualities in some possible future World War III that America might be planning; rather, I hoped that by getting accurate information about this kind of problem I could contribute to the control of these weapons or to their elimination, and to the cause of peace in general. A very simple approach, but it taught me a lot. It meant that that I had to come to grips with the social, ethical, and political reasons why I was doing research of a particular kind. The usual kind of justification which social scientists make for their work— "Well, I'm studying man; everything is grist for my mill because I'm studying man"—would no longer do.

As I have often said, both my wife and I became survivors of Hiroshima by proxy. We became so involved with the people who had undergone the experience, and so committed to making their experience known, that we too shared in that experience. In doing research that has any force I think one has to enter into an empathic relationship with the people one is studying. My having been involved as a researcher in a holocaust of this scale has left me with a lasting imprint that continues to inform all the work I do. That was a fundamental lesson to me about advocacy research, because one cannot be neutral to the subject of the atomic bomb.

My involvement in Vietnam also began in a rather personal way when my wife and I went to Indochina in 1954. The French were leaving then and America was taking over the colonial mission. I remember the

French correspondents often saying to us: "You'll see what will happen to you—the same thing that happened to us. You'll find out." We thought we didn't go in for that kind of colonialism, but we had a lot to learn. My wife had been in Hanoi as a journalist, in 1954, when Ho Chi Minh and the Vietnamese—then the Vietminh—marched in to reclaim their old capital. We experienced a sense of horror as our own country began to violate every principle of humanity—and even of history—in what we have subsequently done in Vietnam. That was the beginning for me of a long involvement in the peace movement and in the teach-ins and the many forms of antiwar protest.

Again, speaking personally, I would say that the intensity of my advocacy took a particular turn with the exposure of My Lai just 2 yr. ago. As soon as My Lai became known—though it wasn't a complete surprise to anybody who had followed what America was doing in Vietnam—it had a very strong personal impact on many people, myself included. I remember feeling emotions of shame and rage. My own rage seemed to have two sources. One was the realization that my own country was responsible for this brutality—rage toward the war makers in power. The second was the shame and guilt—rage toward myself—at somehow not having personally done more, whatever little one can do, to confront or fight or prevent this kind of thing from happening. I also felt a professional response because I immediately sensed that what was going on in My Lai had direct relationship to things I had studied and learned in Hiroshima involving immersion in death and the psychology of the survivor. I felt I had a kind of responsibility to involve myself increasingly, which I did. At the same time I tried to remain sensitive to my own subjective reactions to this involvement. I began to think a lot about war crimes and eventually came together with a lawyer and a historian to edit a book on crimes of war.* In that book we focused particularly on American war crimes in Vietnam. It was through antiwar work that I came to the antiwar veterans, and I would stress both the political and professional avenues which brought me to the work.

During the last several years, as I have looked into the war experience, I learned much about the problems faced by Vietnam veterans. In Decem-

---

*Crimes of War: A legal, political, and psychological inquiry into the responsibility of leaders, citizens, and soldiers for criminal acts in wars, edited by Richard A. Falk, Gabriel Kolko, and Robert Jay Lifton, New York; Random House and Vintage Books, 1971.

ber, 1970, I began to meet with antiwar veterans in sessions that we called rap groups. I also began to interview a number of veterans individually and I spent about 10 hr. interviewing a survivor of My Lai who had refused to shoot. At the same time I was involved in various forms of antiwar work *with* the veterans. But I always felt my major role to be that of an investigator. I saw my own mission as one of deepening our understanding of the war and its consequences, while retaining the kinds of ethical and political commitment that I described in relation to the Hiroshima work. I also got involved in the whole issue of the militarization of American society, but my main focus continued to be on antiwar veterans. I felt that my own previous research and concerns would enable me to make a contribution through work with these men.

There had to be a dialectic in this work between the particularity of the Vietnam war—its very special features—and the recurrent patterns of war in general. There is nothing that occurs with antiwar veterans, or with anybody else in Vietnam, that is related to only one or the other. There is always a dialectic. So in this work I was trying to study the psychological experience of men in this particular war and the relationship of their experience to war mythology in general. This is a very important issue because I think the whole cultural image of war is changing.

Also significant for me as I went on in this work was the exploration of new kinds of relationships one could form while being an investigator and/or a therapist. That's very much what I see the rap groups to be about. In this sort of dual role one learns about the process of change in people whom in our professional roles we call "patients" or "clients," and at the same time one learns something about the possibilities for change in ourselves as professionals. The rap groups revealed something I call the "counterfeit universe" to which psychiatrists and chaplains, our brother spiritual guardians in Vietnam, contribute so much. This all relates to some of the hangups and immoral directions in which psychiatry and psychoanalysis become involved.

In connection with the rap groups I have worked closely with a number of people, including Chaim Shatan, Abby Adams, Betty-Jo League, Peter Lawner, and Florence Volkman Pincus, and there has been a communal effort in ways I will suggest. The rap groups came into being as a result of a letter the head of Vietnam Veterans Against the War wrote to me. He put two requests together in a very significant way. First he said he would like me to do something about the psychological suffering of antiwar veterans who were loathe to go to VA hospitals and clinics. Second, he wanted me to take part in a big public political hearing, the winter soldier investigations. These meetings, being planned for Detroit in early 1971, were intended to expose "the nature of the military policy which results in war crimes and veterans' nightmares," as he put it. He juxtaposed, as inseparable, the political and ethical on the one hand and the psychological on the other. I welcomed this opportunity because I, like many others, have been struggling for ways to bring together my professional with my political and ethical senses. So I agreed to work with the veterans in this combined way. I then called in Hy Shatan, who had worked with me on other related matters. We began meeting with veterans in a kind of antiwar colleagueship in order to evolve a psychological program.

I want to try to give you a feel for some of the hit-or-miss, trial-and-error patterns we evolved as we started to work together. We immediately decided to hold the meetings in the VVAW office. It was a rather ramshackle place—it still is, I think, even after moving to a new and somewhat grander space. It was very uncomfortable physically, but it was interesting how the veterans stuck to their office and wanted to stay on their own turf. However cramped and modest the office was, whenever suggestions were made to move to more comfortable quarters the veterans resisted, offering rationalizations and explanations of one kind or another. In fact, when one group eventually did move to the office of one of the professionals, the group quickly ceased to function. I think that retaining a feeling of one's own turf and keeping an open-ended process are both crucial to this kind of experiment.

We formed a panel of professionals; eventually we had a group of 10 or 15. Most of them were brought together by Hy Shatan in the New York area; many were connected with William Alanson White or New York University. We began to apply ourselves to the problem of what we could do with and for the veterans, and we started to develop a group process which became much more informal than any I had known before. The veterans were not about to assume a "patient" role, and we did not want to give the sessions any kind of medical terminology. So we called the sessions "rap groups" rather than therapy groups. We spoke of ourselves as "professionals" rather than therapists, and the veterans were simply veterans—not patients or clients or anything of that sort. This is a very important aspect of the style of these groups. They have fluid boundaries between professionals and "others" (in this case veterans) that is crucial, I think, for this kind of group experiment.

Even more crucial and fundamental is the constant need we found for the professional to put himself or herself personally on the line. I myself experienced this aspect of the process very vividly. Lots of questions were asked of us, some of them very personal: issues having to do with one's ethical principles and how one does or does not live up to these principles. The question of who we were and are as professionals became just as important as finding out who the veterans were and were becoming. We all knew that these matters were important, and our willingness to share this kind of involvement has been, I think, crucial to the process of the group. Actually we found ourselves welcoming this kind of dialogue.

There are three principles that I began to formulate that seemed to be necessary for this kind of rap group. One is the simple principle of *affinity*. This affinity develops because of a coming together of people who share an overwhelming historical or personal experience, as these vets do, which no one else can fully share. The group begins to pull together to make sense and meaning for the future out of this traumatic experience. A second principle has to do with a kind of being there, a sense of *presence*, of full engagement and integrity, and of openness to mutual impact. One becomes much more than simply a therapist against whom ideas rebound; one has a very active presence in the group. And a third principle is that of *self-generation*. The group itself created much of its own direction and form. Of course, we all had certain inner models of what form the process might take. These models had something to do with the very informal rap groups which the men had already initiated at the office. But their inviting us in was crucial, and the innovations and dynamism that the group has evolved have come from this mutual pattern of self-generation.

I do not want to give the impression that all went smoothly; it didn't. Friendly journalists and others often drifted in. One didn't know who was there, who was a veteran, and who was not. Eventually the veterans took hold and made some rules about who could come in, because, as one of them said: "We felt like monkeys in a zoo." From the beginning the purposes of the group were understood in terms of the twofold principle put forth in the initiating letter: to improve the well-being of the veterans psychologically (a therapeutic purpose), and to convey to the country more of the nature of their experience (a political purpose). The latter goal meant that the currents from the rap groups had to emanate in one way or another to a larger audience, through media that sought us out, and through speaking and writing by the professionals and veterans in the group. The group knew from the beginning that I was an investigator and a writer. I told them that I would write about the group, that I might write a book about it, and that I certainly would write articles about it, as I am now doing. All this they accepted as long as it did not jeopardize one's very immediate sense of being part of the group.

We finally came to an arrangement of having two to four professionals attached to a group, each coming as often as he or she could, which usually meant about two-thirds of the time. There have generally been 7 to 12 veterans at each meeting. The groups have varied enormously in their duration and functioning, but a basic principle has been a kind of fluid coming and going. This applies to both the professionals and the veterans. Many of the veterans live a fluctuating existence; they travel around the country; a number of them, perhaps a majority, do not work regularly. They come in and out of the group. In my group there has been a core of about 20 or 30 veterans whose participation has been both sustained and intense over the year the group has functioned. More than a hundred others have been in and out of the group and have had what we believe to be important experiences, but on an irregular basis. The group has met weekly, first on Saturday afternoons and now Thursday nights, with sessions usually lasting about $3\frac{1}{2}$ hr.

The fluid comings and goings and the open-ended quality of the group have been very important. They lent an aspect of "storefront psychiatry" of a kind that has taken place in other areas. We decided that although the groups would not be open to journalists and broadcasters (we would instead speak to these people after the rap sessions), they were open to anybody who was on active duty or any veteran even if he had not been to Vietnam. Anybody who was faced with the idea of Vietnam as a serviceman or former serviceman was welcome into the group. As this became known people would come in through hearing about the group in one way or another. Sometimes, when old members were actively exploring issues which had built up in the group during previous sessions, the appearance of new people could be jarring. But whenever a newcomer came in he would be greeted warmly. There was a bond of expressed brotherhood in relation to the hated Vietnam experience that the men were confronting in the process, into which the professionals were also drawn as part of a vast social and political movement.

In the three meetings of the professionals that we have had there have been two competing views about what is or should be going on in these groups. Some have taken the position that what we are really doing is group therapy. Essentially it is we, the psychoanalysts and psychiatrists and psychologists, who are giving necessary therapy to the veterans who are, in effect, our patients and clients. In contrast, I have felt that this is an experiment in a "new community" in which we employ elements of group therapy but are basically struggling together toward some new communal sense around a critical stance toward the war and toward elements of society that have contributed to and maintained the war. But obviously both these views are true to some extent. I think that many of the professionals have changed their positions over time and they have tended to move toward the second conception. The veterans generally hold the second position, but they also want some of the therapeutic elements that come with the group therapy tradition.

The tension between these two views has contributed to the development of the groups, but has also led to difficulties. The initial group became too large and split into two, three, and four groups as new ones began and old ones stopped. The group that had split from the original one ceased to function soon after having moved to the office of one of the professionals; and a group that had stopped meeting reinitiated itself in another borough where one or two of the people had moved. We have had inquiries from VVAW offices in various parts of the country asking about starting new groups. There was a somewhat haphazard element in all this—some groups last and some don't. I could go further and illustrate ways in which the principles I have emphasized have been at issue and the manner in which we as professionals have been challenged by the veterans. But I think I have made the essential point about a self-generating group process. I want now to talk about the wider experience of psychiatry in this war and describe why I think this kind of experiment assumes an importance beyond our immediate functioning in these little groups.

The patterns of guilt and rage in antiwar veterans are too complex to describe in full detail here. They are, of course, very strong. I would divide the kinds of guilt that we see regularly in these veterans into three types (though mixtures of these types are common). The first is self-lacerating guilt, which is very destructive. Second, there is what I call "numbed guilt," a static guilt which avoids confrontation. Numbing and guilt often appear together. The third kind, which is the pivotal experience for the extraordinary transformation these men bring about in themselves, is what I call "animating guilt." This guilt gives one access to a source of illumination, as Martin Buber put it. It is activating rather than static.

But the rage in these men, regardless of the form of guilt they experience, is very vivid. It has to do with their being a very special group of survivors who have been into a form of absurd evil—the evil of this war which is not rationalizable and justifiable to them as other wars have been to other veterans. Once they confront the absurdity of that evil they are left with the struggle to overcome guilt and to transform themselves into a position which they can psychologically support.

In working with these men it has been interesting to follow their

attitudes toward chaplains and "shrinks." They seem to have more contempt and more anger toward chaplains and shrinks than toward anybody
else they encountered in the military, including the officers who ordered them
into combat in Vietnam. They tell story after story of absurd situations
involving chaplains who blessed their guns and their ammunition, putting
God on our side. A typical description by a Catholic veteran was this:
"Yes, I did go to confession and say, 'Sure I'm smoking dope; I guess I
blew my state of grace again'; but I didn't say anything about killing."
One confesses in a ritualistic way to small transgressions in order to avoid
confessing the ultimate transgression, that of killing for evil purposes or
for no purpose at all. And there were similar feelings about the false witness,
as I think of it, that chaplains lent themselves to at various ceremonies
for the dead. When one's buddy died the chaplain would sometimes join
in the gung-ho feelings that the buddy's death had to be avenged. There is
a great psychological need for a survivor to find meaning in the deaths
of those near to him, and to overcome his own guilt about remaining alive
by finding some significance in these deaths. The veterans feel that the
chaplains encouraged them to find this significance in glorification of the
nation's mission in Vietnam, which meant, in practice, the killing of more
civilians and the perpetuation of evil. Precisely this form of false witness
contributed greatly to My Lai, though in that case it was born and expressed
by the company commander, who combined a funeral ceremony for a
highly regarded noncommissioned officer killed by a mine with an extra-
vagant "pep talk" about "getting back at them" by "destroying everything
living" in the village. There was a chaplain present who participated in the
ceremony and thereby lent what could be called spiritual legitimacy to that
message.

The attitude toward psychiatry and shrinks is in the same tone. The
men tell stories in the rap groups of disturbing encounters they have had
with psychiatrists in Vietnam or near Vietnam after being evacuated. They
tell how after they become overwhelmed with anxiety, and are unwilling
or unable to return to duty, they are put through what is now sometimes
called "the new psychiatry." This was developed first at the end of World
War II, and then in the Korean War, where, I confess, I participated in it
myself. Now in the Vietnam War one is treated close to duty with a kind of
suppression of symptoms in the expectation of being returned quickly
to one's unit. The three frequently reiterated treatment principles of the
new psychiatry are thus "immediacy, proximity, and expectancy." But the
men in the rap groups know that they were struggling with a situation that
they perceived to be evil. They experienced the psychiatrists as encouraging

the corruptible aspect of themselves. They came for psychiatric help asking for some avenue out of a disturbing situation which pulled them into evil, the easy killing of virtually any Vietnamese in sight. But instead of buttressing that part of the men which still struggled to recognize some of the evil of the situation, the psychiatrists undermined that resistance in them and helped reprogram them for duty. I heard stories of a couple of marines who had been handling corpses, having charge of body bags. Each one came individually to the unit psychiatrist to say, "I just can't take this anymore," and each man was told, "We can help you if you follow our pattern and return to duty; you can again feel yourself to be a man by doing that."

Psychiatry in Vietnam colludes with the most corruptible part of the person—the only part which can be colluded with if the whole Vietnam project is to be maintained. This is a strange ethical place for psychiatry to be. And those who advocate the new psychiatry in the military have a lot to answer for. The new psychiatry has a certain self-enclosed logic to it, but its legitimacy depends on the kind of war it is propping up.

One hears accolades for the new psychiatry based on the claim that few Americans have suffered psychiatric casualties from the war; however, these claims are meaningless unless one asks two basic questions: (1) What happens to these men after they leave combat and return home? (2) What are they helped to adjust to in Vietnam? I would answer that second question by saying that psychiatrists in Vietnam help the GIs adjust to committing war crimes. Whatever their individually humane inclinations, psychiatrists and chaplains in Vietnam contribute to the deepening of what can best be called a "counterfeit universe."

No wonder that GIS are enraged at chaplains and shrinks. The only thing worse than being ordered to perform activities that lead almost inevitably to war crimes or slaughter is to have the situation legitimized by those looked to as spiritual guardians. Hence veterans distrust religion and psychiatry in civilian life, and understandably tend to avoid VA psychiatric clinics. That suspicion was expressed frequently in rap groups and was sometimes directed toward the professionals there. The veterans kept raising questions about authenticity, struggling to extricate themselves from the counterfeit universe of Vietnam and from what they saw to be the reinforcement of that counterfeit universe by chaplains and shrinks.

I have already suggested some of my conclusions from this experience and need not belabor them. Essentially I have been describing an experience which has helped me to bring my social and political perspectives together with my professional one. The professionals working with the antiwar veterans have a sense that there is something very important about these men and something very fundamental going on in their personal struggles. We feel that they have something in common with shamans, medicine men, prophets, and healers who in primitive and religiously based societies go into what is called "the land of death." They enter into an extreme experience in order to survive it and come back to their people with new (or old) wisdom, and with a prediction of possible doom unless that wisdom is acted upon. Our sense of ourselves as professionals is to join in this process and try to contribute to it whatever illumination we can, while helping the men as individuals in ways they seek help. When these men try to return to society through the transformation I have described, they call the process "becoming human again." It is interesting that they do this partly by recognizing belatedly the humanity of the Vietnamese whom they have so brutalized, and then going through four related processes that I shall now suggest as relevant to us as well. First, they undergo a pattern which I call only somewhat facetiously "from John Wayne to 'Country Joe and the Fish.'" It means questioning, mocking, and rejecting, the idea of dying in Vietnam—and ultimately of dying blindly, with reckless male bravado and violence, for any cause. Country Joe and the Fish's song "I'm Fixin' to Die Rag" is already something of a classic, and likely to be remembered as *the* song of the Vietnam War. It is, in fact, extremely popular among troops there, though, as one veteran told me, "It took me a while to *hear* what it was saying." What it was saying, of course, is that the whole idea of dying in Vietnam is totally absurd.

The second step is finding, psychologically speaking, a place to land in this transformation. They often find such a place by adopting a stance of protest and identifying with some part of the counterculture where they begin to find colleagues and cohorts outside of the veterans they have known.

The third and related process is simply learning to feel. Of course these men have enormous problems with intimacy and trust, and learning to feel again is a very significant part of the rap sessions. Finally they struggle to achieve some new formulation of self and world. The survivors of the Hiroshima bomb have also had great struggles in connection with formulation, with giving form and significance to their experience. And for them too both introspection and extrospection are important. They, like the veterans, feel the need to look outside as well as inside themselves for sources of meaning and form.

Perhaps we have a bit of a model here for ourselves. I wonder whether we as professionals are capable of looking at issues of death in our personal and professional existence. Can we look honestly at death in our cultural and personal lives? Can we confront the threat of death in certain aspects of our professional experience, in institutions that no longer seem to be working, as well as the apocalyptic threats in our society in general, whether of destruction of the environment or of nuclear war? Once one has developed some capacity to confront these issues, then one has to confront again the uses to which he puts his professional work. Does one continue prostituting psychiatry for anybody who asks for it, or do we use our professional tradition in the service of making a critique of the whole enterprise of war making and militarism at this point in our history?

Where do *we* land when we begin to change in this way? There is a lot of talk about radical therapy and about therapists as radicals, but it really is a difficult kind of question because we can't very comfortably simply plunge into the radical militancy of youth culture. But we can, in a parallel way, at least join in some form of oppositional commitment in which we can employ our professional tradition to raise fundamental issues about our society and culture.

We too have to move beyond professional technicism and "learn to feel" in all this. We have got into the habit of being "neutral screens" and detached therapists. That part of our tradition still bedevils us. We have to begin to combine our professional skills with a return to the ethical passion that we seem to have lost at many points along the way. And finally, can *we* use the model of ourselves as survivors and begin to shape our lives in new ways—ways that have more exploratory mobility? And in thus reformulating self and world, can we too find a style that combines introspection and extrospection so that we no longer look at society and the historical process as something we call "reality," as a mere backdrop for psychological experience?

In closing I come back to a line of poetry that has haunted me ever since I first heard it, a line I find myself returning to in moments like this. It is a line of Theodore Roethke: "In a dark time the eyes can see." I think that this is a very dark time. Yet, paradoxically and strangely, it is a time of rare opportunity for those of us in the psychological professions—an opportunity to see more in our study of this elusive human being, to feel more, and to do more.

Name Index

Page numbers in italic refer to papers or discussions of papers that are printed in this volume. Thanks are due to Miss Savilla M. Laird for aid in the preparation of the Name Index and the Subject Index.

272

Subject Index